VEGAN
MEAL PREP

Tasty Plant-Based Whole Foods Recipes
With a 30-Day Time-Saving Meal Plan

By Jules Neumann
Version 3.1
Published by HMPL Publishing
Get to know your publisher and related work at
happyhealthygreen.life

Introduction

Achieve your health and fitness goals with a simple discipline called prepping meals, or meal prepping. By managing and monitoring your nutrition, you'll get in shape, save hours of time, and avoid waste. Cook your meals in bulk in advance, and simply eat when it's time to eat. Kiss fast food and cravings goodbye and spend your time where it truly matters – outside of the kitchen.

Vegan meal-prep will teach you the art of forming life-long healthy habits; learn how to buy ingredients in advance, understand your body's needs, and prepare a large number of meals in a single kitchen session. You'll experience less stress and foster not only your physical, but also your mental and emotional wellbeing. On top of that you'll feel confident knowing exactly what nutrition you will consume tomorrow.

Start reading the information and then move on to prepping the easiest meals first. You'll benefit from the included 30-day meal plan that comes with this book, learning how to calculate macronutrients and calories. Ultimately, this will help you to become the master of your own physique.

This book will guide you through the process of planning, prepping, tracking, and storing meals. As you get better at these tasks, you'll have more and more free time for your real life. You'll start to love your fridge and freezer and dramatically reduce your trips to the grocery store or restaurants.

Table of Contents

Lunch Recipes 86

Dinner Recipes 112

Disclaimer

The recipes provided in this report are for informational purposes only and are not intended to provide dietary advice. A medical practitioner should be consulted before making any changes in your diet. Additionally, recipe cooking times may require adjustment depending on age and quality of appliances. Readers are strongly urged to take all precautions to ensure ingredients are fully cooked in order to avoid the dangers of foodborne viruses. The recipes and suggestions provided in this book are solely the opinion of the author. The author and publisher do not take any responsibility for any consequences that may result due to following the instructions provided in this book.

About Us

Welcome to the reader's circle of happyhealthygreen.life. You can subscribe to our newsletter using this link:

http://happyhealthygreen.life/vegan-newsletter

By subscribing to our newsletter, you will receive the latest vegan recipes, tips about health & nutrition and plant-based cooking articles that make your mouth water, right in your inbox. We also offer you a unique opportunity to read future vegan cookbooks for absolutely free...

Get your hands on free vegan recipes and instant access to 'The Vegan Cookbook'. Subscribe to the vegan newsletter and grab your free copy here at:

http://happyhealthygreen.life/vegan-newsletter

Enter your email address to get instant access. Support veganism and say NO to animal cruelty!

We don't like spam and understand you don't like spam either. We'll email you no more than 2 times per week.

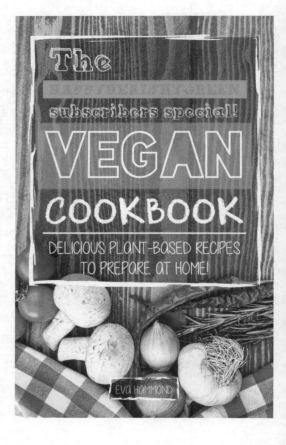

What is Veganism?

Veganism is not just a diet; it is a lifestyle choice that requires a fair amount of thought and can be based on health, ethics, or religious beliefs.

A vegan diet is plant-based. The difference between the vegetarian and vegan diets is that while vegetarians only eliminate meat, vegans cut out all animal products. This includes dairy, eggs and food ingredients and supplements derived from animals- such as gelatin, albumin, and squalene. (Though ovo-vegetarians eat eggs but not dairy, while lacto-vegetarians consume dairy but not eggs.)

Ethical considerations that may lead a person to veganism include desiring not to support a practice that harms or kills animals or concern for the environment. People also become vegan for health reasons—many believe that the human body was not designed to consume animal products. For example, animal products are high in saturated fats and contain animal hormones that may cause imbalances in humans. Lactose intolerance and concern over harmful animal pathogens and bi-products are also common. In addition to various harmful components that are naturally found in animal products, many products also undergo processing treatments in production and end up containing high concentrations of preservatives.

Although a vegan diet provides most required nutrients, extra care must be taken to ensure that some nutrients such as amino acids and vitamin B12, which are more readily available in animal products than in plants, are consumed in sufficient quantities.

Goals

We often hear people complaining about wanting to have more time to achieve more, but also to do the things they enjoy, such as spending time with friends and family, reading, or just relaxing. Preparing you meals will give you more time to do these things and you will save more money and become a better, healthier version of yourself. Learning the art of meal prep is a worthy investment!

Saving time

Preparing your meals in advance for the week means no more worrying about what you are going to eat for breakfast, lunch, and dinner on a daily basis. You won't have to tire yourself out at the end of the day browsing recipes, shopping, washing, chopping, and cooking. Once you have gotten into the habit of thinking ahead and preparing, you will find that grocery shopping becomes much less laborious and time-consuming. With this system, you only have to devote one day of planning per week, allowing more free time than you've ever had before.

Saving money

The notion that fast food is cheap and that healthy food is a luxury for the wealthy is a misconception. Preparing healthy, home-cooked meals can actually save you money. If you are not convinced, list the cost of each ingredient that goes into your next home-cooked meal and compare the total to the price of the same dish at your local restaurant.

Healthy meals in restaurants are extremely costly. The amount you would spend on one healthy meal in a restaurant is the equivalent to a weekly trip to the grocery store can last you several days. The average cost of each meal prepared at home is five to eight dollars/euros, which is less than you would spend buying those unhealthy fast food meals that are commonly believed to be "cheap".

Eating healthy and losing weight

Through preparing and storing meals, you will also be able to learn how to control your portion intake, since you will be using containers made up of compartments intended for the separation of meal components into the desired portions. When dividing portions, there are a number of aspects to consider, including calorie count and macronutrient proportions. Taking in a lower number of calories will help you shed some weight. The number of daily calories required in order to lose weight are shown in the percentage-based caloric deficit table below. These will not be empty calories as the vegan meals you prepare will be packed with nutrition to increase performance, brainpower and general health.

Be sure to note the nutritional information of each meal on the storage containers you use, as well as the weight of the portion. Once your containers are labeled, you can estimate the daily amount of calories and macros you will be taking in. To make it easy sticking to the caloric deficit required to achieve your goals. Calculating your daily caloric needs will be explained in the subchapter "Counting calories".

Calorie Maintenance Levels Per Day	20% Caloric Deficit
1600 calories	320 calories below the maintenance level (1280 calories on a daily basis)
1800 calories	360 calories below the maintenance level (1440 calories on a daily basis)
2000 calories	400 calories below the maintenance level (1600 calories on a daily basis)
2500 calories	500 calories below the maintenance level (2000 calories on a daily basis)
3000 calories	600 calories below the maintenance level (2400 calories on a daily basis)
4000 calories	800 calories below the maintenance level (3200 calories on a daily basis)

Macros and Micros

Macronutrients or "macros" is the name given to three groups of energy-dense nutrients which make up the most basic components of our diets: carbohydrates, fats, and proteins. In addition to acting as fuel for bodily energy, they facilitate many of our bodies' functions and are broken down by our digestive system for use in bodily structures. Each macronutrient provides us with the following number of calories:

- *1 g protein = 4 calories*
- *1 g carb = 4 calories*
- *1 g fat = 9 calories*

Counting Calories

When preparing your meals, you will need to calculate their macronutrient breakdown and how many calories each meal contains. The included meal-plan provides this already if you choose to follow or pick days to eat from the 30-day meal plan. To benefit from this process, you need to know how much you need to eat each day. That's why daily caloric needs; also known as basal metabolic rate, is essential for keeping track of your daily macro intake. How to calculate your specific needs is explained in the following paragraph.

This is the formula you need to use to calculate basal metabolic rate (BMR):
- **Men:** BMR = (9.99 x weight in kilograms) + (6.25 x height in centimeters) - 4.92 x age in years + 5.
- **Women:** BMR = (9.99 x weight in kilograms) + (6.25 x height in centimeters) - (4.92 x age in years) - 161.
- **Multiply the BMR number with the activity factor that fits your lifestyle.** With no exercise, your activity factor is 1.2. Exercise one to three times a week and your activity factor is 1.375. If you engage in exercise three to five times per week, the activity factor is 1.55. For heavy exercise, six to seven times a week, the activity factor is 1.725 and in case of an athlete or heavy training sessions and/or have a physically demanding job, your activity factor is 1.9. The number derived from this second calculation is the number of calories (kcal) required for maintaining a healthy weight.

Lowering your carb and fat intakes will allow you to burn fat more efficiently. For some body builders, a *carb to protein to fat* intake ratio of 50:25:25 is ideal. Once you have achieved your goals and wish to simply maintain your body weight, you need to focus on stabilizing your caloric intake with at least 15-20% of your calories coming from protein.

The following is a breakdown of how to achieve the 50:25:25 ratio on a 2000-calorie diet:
- 50% carbohydrates: 2000 x 50% = 1000 calories per day. To determine the grams needed, divide 1000 by 4 to get 250 grams of carbohydrates required on a daily basis.
- 25% protein: 2000 x 25% = 500 calories per day. Divide 500 calories by 4 to get 125 g of protein needed on a daily basis.
- 25% fat: 2000 x 25% = 500 calories per day. Divide 500 calories by 9 to get ~55.6 g of fat needed on a daily basis.

Protein

Protein is vital to the proper functioning of all living things. The basic molecules that make up proteins are amino acids, also known as "the building blocks of life". Amino acids compose many of the body's structures including nails, muscle, skin and hair. Some sources of vegan protein include tempeh, beans, quinoa, lentils, raw arugula, russet potatoes, raw collard greens, raw broccoli, raw spinach, boiled water chestnuts, boiled artichokes, boiled sweet corn and raw kale.

The table below shows the protein sources and their macronutrient breakdowns:

Food	Serving	Metric	Fats(g)	Carbs(g)	Fiber(g)	Protein(g)	Net Carbs(g)
Edamame	100g	100g	9	8.4	6	18.2	2.4
Lentils	100g	100g	0.4	20.1	7.9	9	12.2
White Beans	100g	100g	0.4	25.1	6.3	9.7	18.8
Cranberry Beans (Roman Beans)	100g	100g	0.5	24.5	8.6	9.3	15.9
Split Peas	100g	100g	0.4	21.1	8.3	8.3	12.8
Pinto Beans	100g	100g	0.7	26.2	9	9	17.2

Food	Serving	Metric	Fats(g)	Carbs(g)	Fiber(g)	Protein(g)	Net Carbs(g)
Kidney Beans	100g	100g	0.5	22.8	6.4	8.7	16.4
Black Beans	100g	100g	0.5	23.7	8.7	8.9	15
Navy Beans	100g	100g	0.6	26.1	10.5	8.2	15.6
Lima Beans	100g	100g	0.3	23.6	5.4	6.8	18.2
Cornmeal (Grits)	100g	100g	3.6	76.9	7.3	8.1	69.6
Kamut	100g	100g	0.8	27.6	4.3	5.7	23.3
Teff, cooked	100g	100g	0.7	19.9	2.8	3.9	17.1
Quinoa	100g	100g	1.9	21.3	2.8	4.4	18.5
Couscous, cooked	1 oz.	86g	0.1	20	1.2	3.3	18.8
Oatmeal	100g	100g	1.5	12	1.7	2.5	10.3
Buckwheat Groats	100g	100g	0.6	19.9	2.7	3.4	17.2
Millet	100g	100g	1	23.7	1.3	3.5	22.4
Artichokes	100g	100g	0.2	10.5	5.4	10.5	5.1
Green Peas	100g	100g	0.2	15.6	5.5	5.4	10.1
Soybean Sprouts	½ cup	35g	2.3	3.3	0.4	4.6	3
Yellow Corn Sweet	100g	100g	1.4	18.7	2	3.3	16.7
Brussels Sprouts	½ cup	78g	0.4	5.5	2	2	3.5
Button Mushrooms	100g	100g	0.3	4	1.8	3.6	2.2
Broccoli	½ cup	78g	0.3	5.6	2.6	1.9	3
Guavas	100g	100g	1	14.3	5.4	2.6	8.9
Apricots	100g	100g	0.4	11.1	2	1.4	9.1
Kiwifruit	100g	100g	0.5	14.7	3	1.1	11.7
Blackberries	100g	100g	0.5	9.6	5.3	1.4	4.3
Oranges	100g	100g	0.1	11.8	2.4	0.9	9.4
Cantaloupe Melons	100g	100g	0.2	8.2	0.9	0.8	7.3

Food	Serving	Metric	Fats(g)	Carbs(g)	Fiber(g)	Protein(g)	Net Carbs(g)
Hemp Seed	1 oz.	28g	13.8	2.5	1.1	9	1.3
Pumpkin Seeds	1 oz.	28g	13.9	4.2	1.8	8.5	2.3
Peanuts	1 oz.	28g	14.1	6	2.4	6	3.7
Pistachio Nuts	1 oz.	28g	13	8	2.9	6	5.1
Sunflower Seeds	1 oz.	28g	14.1	4.3	2.6	5.5	1.8
Pine Nuts	1 oz.	28g	19.4	3.7	1.1	3.9	2.7
Chickpeas	1 cup	164g	4.2	45	12.5	14.5	7.9
Amaranth	1 cup	28g	0.1	1.1	0	0.1	1.1

Amino acids are also involved in many of the body's chemical reactions, as they are the basic components of enzymatic structures and other chemical molecules. This ultimately means that they regulate mood, growth, and tissue repair, as they control the buildup and breakdown of complex molecules.

There are 20 amino acids, 9 of which are essential and 11 of which are non-essential. Essential amino acids are those which must be derived from the diet. Plant products do not contain all of the required essential amino acids in large amounts, so vegans need to be vigilant about tracking protein intake from various "incomplete" protein sources. When combined, these foods can cover an individual's full amino acid requirements. Of course, this does not mean that you must eat sources of all the amino acids within the same meal at the same time. You can combine a variety of legumes, nuts, unrefined grains, seeds, and whole vegetables over the course of a week to meet your needs.

The nine essential amino acids are leucine, lysine, tryptophan, isoleucine, histidine, valine, methionine, phenylalanine and threonine.

Beans and legumes contain high levels of lysine but are lacking in methionine. Examples include kidney beans, peanuts, peas, black beans, lentils, and garbanzo beans. These sources can therefore be combined with grains such as rice which are high in methionine.

Leafy greens like spinach, kale, broccoli and romaine lettuce are high in leucine, valine, phenylalanine, and lysine.

A couple of exceptional plant foods are soy and quinoa, which contain a great balance of amino acids. Soy contains all nine essential amino acids, making it a complete protein source.

The following list is a breakdown of the nine essential amino acids, their functions, sources and daily requirements:

Note: daily requirements of amino acid are not extremely strict, since it's easy to get enough on a vegan diet with enough variety.

Lysine
Function: tissue growth, carnitine production
Requirements: 2000 - 3500 mg
Sources: beans, hemp, legumes (chickpeas and lentils), almonds, watercress, parsley, chia seeds, avocados, cashews and spirulina

Leucine (branched-chain amino acid or BCAA)
Functions: muscle growth and maintenance, blood sugar regulation
Requirements: 2000 - 3000 mg
Sources: peas, avocados, raisins, seaweed, pumpkin, whole grain rice, watercress, sesame seeds, turnip greens, kidney beans, figs, dates, blueberries, soy, apples, sunflower seeds, olives and bananas

Isoleucine

Functions: production of hemoglobin, energy production, muscle tissue repair

Requirements: 2000 - 3200 mg

Sources: brown rice, lentils, cabbage, rye, cashews, almonds, soy, sunflower seeds, sesame seeds, oats, beans, chia seeds, spinach, hemp seeds, pumpkin, pumpkin seeds, cranberries, blueberries, apples, quinoa and kiwi fruit

Methionine

Functions: cartilage formation

Requirements: 1050 - 1500 mg

Sources: whole grain rice, seaweed, beans, sunflower seeds, chia seeds, Brazil nuts, hemp seeds, oats, wheat, figs, onions, cacao, legumes and raisins

Phenylalanine (converted to tyrosine by the body)

Requirements: up to 8g (should be avoided by pregnant women)

Functions: hormone production precursor

Sources: quinoa, almonds, figs, leafy greens, spirulina, beans, rice, pumpkin, avocados, peanuts, most berries, raisins, olives and seeds

Threonine

Functions: immunity, nervous system maintenance

Requirements: 1050-1500 mg

Sources: soybeans, sesame seeds, chia seeds, watercress, pumpkin, leafy greens, spirulina, hemp seeds, raisins, sunflower seeds, almonds, avocados, figs, quinoa and wheat

Tryptophan

Functions: mood regulation, sleep cycle regulation, circulation support, enzyme production, metabolism and central nervous system regulation

Requirements: 280 – 350 mg

Sources: leafy greens, mushrooms, beans, figs, winter squash, oats, hemp seeds, chia seeds, seaweed, beans, beets, parsley, asparagus, all lettuces, avocados, celery, carrots, chickpeas, peppers, lentils, onions, oranges, bananas, apples, spinach, soybeans, pumpkin, watercress, sweet potatoes, quinoa and peas

Valine

Functions: growth and repair of muscles

Requirements: 1600-2800 mg

Sources: soy, peanuts, chia seeds, whole grains, beans, legumes, broccoli, sesame seeds, spinach, cranberries, oranges, hemp seeds, avocados, apples, figs, blueberries, apricots, and sprouted grains and seeds

Histidine

Functions: transportation of neurotransmitters

Requirements: 650 – 800 mg

Sources: wheat, beans, cantaloupe, hemp seeds, legumes, rice, rye, seaweed, chia seeds, potatoes, cauliflower, buckwheat and corn

Fats

Over the past three decades, it has been drilled into our minds that fats are bad. Period. However, the truth of the matter is that the body needs fats. For one, we need fat to absorb certain fat-soluble vitamins like A, D, E and K. Without fat, the body is not able to absorb those much-needed vitamins. Additionally, we need fat for healthy skin and hair as well as a protective insulator.

Your body is unable to produce essential fatty acids, so it is critical that you consume good fat sources. These essential fats help with numerous body processes like regulating blood pressure, protecting organs and brain development functions.

Consuming unsaturated fats is your best bet. Unsaturated fats are in a liquid state and generally come from plant sources. Saturated fats are solid and generally come from animal sources. Trans fats are a third major fat. These fats are often produced by companies trying to increase the shelf life of their products. Trans fats are unsaturated fats that are turned into saturated fats by hydrogenizing the unsaturated fat. Needless to say, trans fats are super bad and should be avoided.

Plant-based oils are a great vegan source of unsaturated fats. Butters like cocoa butter and coconut cream are also great sources of healthy vegan fats. There have been studies stating coconut oil is "overrated" as it only temporarily aids your body's nutritional levels. In fact, while coconut oil may claim to decrease LDL levels (your "bad" cholesterol levels) it actually eventually adds to your LDL levels in the long run. As a result, while many recipes lean towards the use of coconut oil, remember that any oil of your choice works just as well. These include sunflower oil, flax seed oil and olive oil, which give your body a well-balanced array of fats.

Omega 3-6-9

Fatty acids are vital for your body's functions, from your respiratory and circulatory systems to your brain and other vital organs. Ultimately, while the body does produce fatty acids such as the Omega-9 fatty acid on its, there are two essential fatty acids (EFAs) it cannot produce: Omega-3 and Omega-6.

The Omega-3 fatty acid is responsible for aiding in brain function as well as preventing cardiovascular disease. This fatty acid prevents asthma, certain cancers, arthritis, high cholesterol, blood pressure and so on. Many say that our dosage of Omega-3 can be satisfied by consuming fatty fish such as salmon however, it's a great misconception that vegans lack this vital nutrient due to not consuming fatty-flesh foods. While Omega-3 is most popularly taken from fish, it has a plethora of vegan sources as well, including green vegetables, chia seed oil, flaxseed oils, raw walnuts and hempseed oil to name a few!

The Omega-6 fatty acid is responsible for many of the benefits mentioned above when consumed with Omega-3. Omega-6 can be found in seeds, nuts, green veggies and oils, such as olive oil. The trick is to consume the right levels of these nutrients; you should be consuming double the amount of Omega-6 fatty acid as the Omega-3 or the benefits of these EFAs may actually be cancelled. The world has become victim to fast food and frozen pre-made dishes that have dangerously high amounts of Omega-6; but following a whole foods based diet can ensure your health as you get balanced amounts of each and every nutrient.

The Omega-9 fatty acid is a non-essential fatty acid which the body can produce. Although the body will only produce this fatty acid once there are appropriate levels of both Omega-3 and Omega-6, thus making it dependent on the consumption of the two fatty acids the body cannot produce. If you do not have appropriate amounts of Omega-3 and Omega-6, then you can get additional Omega-9 from your diet (since your body wouldn't be producing it in this case). Omega-9 can be found naturally in avocados, nuts, chia seed oil and olive oil.

Carbs

Carbohydrates are the human body's main energy source and are classed into two groups: simple and complex. Simple carbohydrates are low in nutrients and fiber and are easily broken down into glucose to generate energy. Complex carbohydrates consist of long chains of monosaccharides which take longer to be broken down. Unlike simple carbohydrates, they contain fiber (which keeps you satiated longer after a meal), minerals and vitamins. Complex carbohydrate plant sources include whole grains, lentils, legumes, beans, sweet potatoes and cruciferous.

The Glycemic Index (GI) is a scale used to rank carbohydrates according to the rise of glucose levels in the blood after consumption. High GI carbs release glucose into the blood very rapidly, commonly known as blood sugar spikes. These blood sugar spikes caused by simple carbs should be avoided and can eventually be the cause of diabetes type 2. Complex carbs release glucose slowly because of a low GI (less than 55). Complex carbs are helpful in keeping a stable blood sugar level and should be a staple in your diet.

Micronutrient Intake

Micronutrients (vitamins and minerals) play important roles in most of the body's functions. Vitamins fall into two categories: water-soluble vitamins (C and B complex) and fat-soluble vitamins (A, D, E & K) – *see chart below*. Water-soluble vitamins are held in the body for up to three days and therefore need to be replaced regularly throughout the diet while fat-soluble vitamins can be stored in the liver for up to a year.

On a vegan diet, particular attention needs to be paid to vitamin D, calcium and vitamin B12. Vitamin B12, which plays a vital role in the procession of oxygen-carrying red blood cells, is predominantly found in animal products. Based on recommendations, an adult should consume 2.4mcg of vitamin B12 per day. On a vegan diet it would be wise to supplement and be vigilant about consuming foods such as B12-fortified cereals. Please talk to your nutritionist or dietician about the best way to supplement. Tracking your micro nutrient intake can easily be done by using macronutrient tracking apps that include counting daily intake of vitamins and minerals.

Good plant sources of calcium include leafy greens such as collards and kale, as well as plant-based milk alternatives like soy, almond, rice, or hemp milk. Vitamin D sources include portobello and shiitake mushrooms, as well as fortified milk alternatives. Though the best source of vitamin D is, of course, sunlight, if you live in a predominantly cloudy region of the world, it's a good idea to supplement.

DAILY NEEDS OF MICRONUTRIENTS

Micronutrient	Recommended Dietary Allowance
Calcium	1200 mg
Phosphorus	700 mg
Magnesium	400 mg for men and 310 mg for women
Potassium	4700 mg
Sodium	1500 mg

Micronutrient	Recommended Dietary Allowance
Chloride	2300 mg
Iron	8 mg for men and 18 mg for women
Zinc	11 mg for men, 8 mg for women
Copper	900 µg
Iodine	150 µg
Manganese	2.3 mg for men, 1.8 mg for women
Vitamin A	900 µg for men, 700 µg for women
Vitamin D	15 µg
Vitamin E	15 mg
Vitamin K	120 µg for men, 90 µg for women
Vitamin C	90 mg for men, 75 mg for women
Thiamine (B1)	1.2 mg for men, 1.1 mg for women
Riboflavin (B2)	1.3 mg for men, 1.1 mg for women
Niacin (B3)	16 mg for men, 14 mg for women
Pantothenic acid (B5)	1.3 mg
Pyridoxine (B6)	1.3 mg
Biotin (B7)	30 µg
Folic acid (B9)	400 µg
Cobalamin/Vitamin B12	2.4 µg

Nutrient rich vegan foods

NUTS & SEEDS

Bite-sized nuts and seeds are a convenient and portable snack option. They are packed with savory flavor and can be difficult to stop eating once you start! As they are calorie-dense, it is best to limit your consumption of these little delights, particularly those that are high in carbohydrates such as chestnuts, pistachios and cashews.

The table below illustrates a breakdown of the macronutrient components of different nuts. The serving size has been set to 1 ounce.

Food	Serving	Metric	Fats(g)	Carbs(g)	Fiber(g)	Protein(g)	Net Carbs(g)
Chai seed	1 oz.	28g	9	12	11	4	1
Pecan	1 oz.	28g	20	4	3	3	1
Flax Seed	1 oz.	28g	12	8	7	5	1
Brazil Nut	1 oz.	28g	19	4	2	4	2
Hazelnut	1 oz.	28g	17	5	3	4	2
Walnut	1 oz.	28g	18	4	2	4	2
Coconut, Unsweetened	1 oz.	28g	18	7	5	2	2
Macadamia Nut	1 oz.	28g	21	4	2	2	2
Almond	1 oz.	28g	15	5	3	6	2
Almond Flour	1 oz.	28g	14	6	3	6	3
Pumpkin Seed	1 oz.	28g	6	4	1	10	3
Sesame Seed	1 oz.	28g	14	7	3	5	4
Sunflower Seed	1 oz.	28g	14	7	3	6	4

GREENS

Food	Serving	Metric	Fats(g)	Carbs(g)	Fiber(g)	Protein(g)	Net Carbs(g)
Endive	2 oz.	56g	0	2	2	1	0
Butter Head Lettuce	2 oz.	56g	0	1	0.5	1	0.5
Chicory	2 oz.	56g	0	2.5	2	1	0.5
Beet Greens	2 oz.	56g	0	2.5	2	1	0.5
Bok Choy	2 oz.	56g	0	1	0.5	1	0.5
Alfalfa Sprouts	2 oz.	56g	0	2	1	2	1
Spinach	2 oz.	56g	0	2	1	1.5	1
Swiss Chard	2 oz.	56g	0	2	1	1	1
Arugula	2 oz.	56g	0	2	1	1.5	1
Celery	2 oz.	56g	0	2	1	0.5	1
Chives	2 oz.	56g	0	2.5	1.5	2	1
Collard Greens	2 oz.	56g	0	3	2	1.5	1
Romaine	2 oz.	56g	0	2	1	1	1
Asparagus	2 oz.	56g	0	2	1	1	1
Eggplant	2 oz.	56g	0	3	2	0.5	1
Radishes	2 oz.	56g	0	2	1	0.5	1
Tomatoes	2 oz.	56g	0	2	1	0.5	1
White mushrooms	2 oz.	56g	0	2	0.5	2	1.5
Cauliflower	2 oz.	56g	0	3	1.5	1	1.5
Cucumber	2 oz.	56g	0	2	0.5	0.5	1.5
Dill pickles	2 oz.	56g	0	2	0.5	0.5	1.5

Food	Serving	Metric	Fats(g)	Carbs(g)	Fiber(g)	Protein(g)	Net Carbs(g)
Bell Green Pepper	2 oz.	56g	0	2.5	1	0.5	1.5
Cabbage	2 oz.	56g	0	3	1	1	2
Fennel	2 oz.	56g	0	4	2	1	2
Broccoli	2 oz.	56g	0	3.5	1.5	1.5	2
Green Beans	2 oz.	56g	0	4	2	1	2
Bamboo Shoots	2 oz.	56g	0	3	1	1.5	2

FRUITS

Food	Serving	Metric	Fats(g)	Carbs(g)	Fiber(g)	Protein(g)	Net Carbs(g)
Rhubarb	2 oz.	56g	0	2.5	1	1	1.5
Lemon Juice	1 oz.	28g	0	2	0	0	2
Lime Juice	1 oz.	28g	0	2	0	0	2
Raspberries	2 oz.	56g	0	7	4	1	3
Blackberries	2 oz.	56g	0	6	3	1	3
Strawberries	2 oz.	56g	0	4	1	0	3

PROTEIN RICH VEGAN FOODS

Amino acids result from the breakdown of protein by the body after it is ingested and go on to be used for tissue growth and repair. As proteins take longer to be digested than carbohydrates, they provide higher levels of satiety. Protein also contains fewer calories. Some good vegan options are shown in the table below.

Food	Serving	Metric	Fats(g)	Carbs(g)	Fiber(g)	Protein(g)	Net Carbs(g)
Tofu	100g	100g	9	4	2	16	2
Pumpkin Seed	1 oz.	28g	6	4	1	10	3
Almond	1 oz.	28g	15	5	3	6	2
Flax Seed	1 oz.	28g	12	8	7	5	1
Chia Seed	1 oz.	28g	9	12	11	4	1
Brazil Nut	1 oz.	28g	19	4	2	4	2
Hazelnut	1 oz.	28g	17	5	3	4	2
Walnut	1 oz.	28g	18	4	2	4	2
Pecan	1 oz.	28g	20	4	3	3	1
Unsweetened Coconut	1 oz.	28g	18	7	5	2	2
Macadamia Nut	1 oz.	28g	21	4	2	2	2

FAT RICH VEGAN FOODS

The healthy fats, mono-unsaturated and poly-unsaturated fats, are a vital part of our diet. They contain what is known as "good cholesterol", or more accurately, high-density lipoproteins (HDL) and very high-density lipoproteins (VHDL). They keep your blood lipid profile in check and in reducing the negative effects of "bad cholesterol" on the cardiovascular system. As a general rule, plant fats are considered to be healthy. Avoid foods which contain trans fats.

Food	Serving	Metric	Fats(g)	Carbs(g)	Fiber(g)	Protein(g)	Net Carbs(g)
Avocado oil	1 oz.	28g	28	0	0	0	0
Cocoa butter	1 oz.	28g	28	0	0	0	0
Coconut oil	1 oz.	28g	28	0	0	0	0
Flaxseed oil	1 oz.	28g	28	0	0	0	0
Macadamia oil	1 oz.	28g	28	0	0	0	0
MCT oil	1 oz.	28g	28	0	0	0	0
Olive oil	1 oz.	28g	28	0	0	0	0
Coconut cream	1 oz.	28g	10	2	1	1	1
Olives, green	1 oz.	28g	4	1	1	0	0
Avocado	1 oz.	28g	4	2	2	1	0

Labelling food

Keeping organized and labelling your prepared food will save you a lot of time and stress. You don't want to have to endlessly open and close containers to find what you're looking for. Labels will also help you keep track of what you have so that you can buy more ingredients when necessary.

When putting containers in the freezer, be sure to use freezer-friendly labels so that they will not lose adhesiveness in the low temperature and will remain legible. Other labelling materials that can come in handy include permanent or dry erase markers, sticky notes, stickers, date labels and transparent adhesive tape.

When labelling be sure to include:
- The date the food was prepared on
- Meal name and/or description (recipes included in this book)
- Expiration date
- Macronutrient breakdown

FOOD STORAGE AND CONTAINERS

Common food-storing methods include:

1. **Chilling and freezing** – storing food at lower temperatures maintains its freshness and nutritious value for longer.
2. **Drying food** – dehydrating foods (sun drying, air-drying, oven drying and smoking) keeps food from going bad as bacteria cannot thrive without moisture.
3. **Canning** – sealing food in airtight containers also stops bacteria/fungi from multiplying, as they require oxygen.
4. **Pickling** – storing food in vinegar and salt mixtures is a common method for preserving fresh food.

When choosing an appropriate container, factors such as portion size, storage time, fridge/freezer space and dimensions should be taken into consideration. Being familiar with your storage capacity will ensure that you are not wasting ingredients and buying things you cannot keep. Utilizing containers with different sections will prevent cross-contamination of the different elements of your prepared meals and improve their aesthetics.

Check to make sure that the containers you buy are bisphenol (BPA) -free. This chemical is detrimental to health. Clear containers will enable you to identify your meals more easily when they are stacked. Bento boxes and other washable/reusable containers are best.

For longer storage periods, a vacuum sealer may also be useful.

Some typical food storage containers include:

1. **Polycarbonate containers:** transparent boxes that allow for easy stacking and identification. They are shatterproof and have airtight lids.
2. **Polypropylene containers:** resistant to temperatures between -40 and 70 degrees Celsius. They are stackable, have airtight lids and are BPA-free.
3. **Stainless steel containers:** temperature resistant but not suitable for the microwave.
4. **Glass container:** quality containers that are easy to keep clean. They are resistant to temperatures, stackable and suitable for the microwave
5. **Ingredient bins:** used to store bulk foods like grains.

WAYS TO HEAT YOUR STORED FOOD

You will need to reheat some of your prepared meals before eating them. Here are the best ways for this to be done:

1. **On the stove**: place your food in a saucepan and heat it thoroughly.
2. **In the oven**: place in a heat resistant container or baking dish at a low temperature so that the outside of the food is not burned.
3. **The microwave:** an option which will save you a lot of time, making meal prepping easier. If you choose to use a microwave, ensure that you use microwave safe containers.

Chafing tables, steam tables and slow cookers are not recommended. If food is exposed to a certain temperature (between 4.4 and 60 degrees centigrade), bacteria proliferation can occur, leading to food poisoning.

Soaking methods and cooking recipes for vegan staple foods

A few vegan ingredients come up time again in vegan recipes and are good to have on hand. These ingredients are ideal for adding texture, flavor, fiber and protein to your meals. Amongst them are beans, grains, nuts, seeds, oil, dried fruits and vegetables. Some of these (seeds, nuts and fruits) are also great to have as snacks.

SOAKING

Beans, lentils and split peas are rich in protein and fiber and are incorporated into many vegan recipes. However, they require soaking before cooking in order to be softened. This reduces the cooking time needed and helps digestion. Many of the 'anti-nutrients' found in beans are water-soluble, so they're removed during soaking. Anti-nutrients prevent nutrient absorption in the gastrointestinal tract. An alternative to soaking is sprouting. These methods are explained in the tables below.

OVERNIGHT SOAK

Leaving beans, lentils and legumes in a pot of water overnight (at least 8 hours) is the most effective way to soak. Use roughly 10 cups of water for every pound of dry beans (roughly 2 cups). Required soaking times are shown in the table below.

HOT SOAK

This is the quickest soaking method. Fill up a pot large enough to accommodate your beans or legumes with water. Add about 10 cups for each pound (roughly 2 cups) of dry beans, or make sure beans/legumes are covered with an excess of about 1 inch of water. Bring the water to a boil and allow it to simmer for about 3 minutes. Remove the pot from the heat, cover and allow it to sit for 1 to 4 hours.

RINSING

After soaking, drain the water from the pot and rinse the beans or legumes once or twice with fresh, cool water. This will wash off the indigestible sugars and anti-nutrients.

BOILING

After soaking and rinsing, fill a large pot to accommodate your beans or legumes with an excess of 1 inch of water. Lower the heat to reach a medium boil. Partially cover the pot with a lid. Cooking times vary according to the kind of bean or legume used and are shown below.

Cannallini, white kidney and red beans need boiling to get rid of poison.

Optionally, add acidic ingredients like lemon juice, vinegar or wine after cooking and draining the beans to prevent them from becoming tender.

SOAKING AND COOKING TIME PER BEAN OR LEGUME

(Per 1 cup)	Soak Time	Cooking Time	Yield (in cups)
Azuki Beans	4 hrs.	45-55 min.	3
Anasazi Beans	4-8 hrs.	60 min.	2-1/4
Black Beans	4 hrs.	60-90 min.	2-1/4
Black-eyed Peas	-	60 min.	2
Cannellini Beans	8-12 hrs.	60 min.	2
Fava Beans	8-12 hrs.	40-50 min.	1-2/3
Chickpeas	6-8 hrs.	1-3 hrs.	2
Great Northern Beans	8-12 hrs.	1-1/2 hrs.	2-2/3

(Per 1 cup)	Soak Time	Cooking Time	Yield (in cups)
Green Split Peas	-	45 min.	2
Yellow Split Peas	-	60-90 min.	2
Green Peas, whole	8-12 hrs.	1-2 hrs.	2
Kidney Beans	6-8 hrs.	60 min.	2-1/4
Lentils, brown	8-12 hrs.	45-60 min.	2-1/4
Lentils, green	8-12 hrs.	30-45 min.	2
Lentils, red or yellow	8-12 hrs.	20-30 min.	2 to 2-1/2
Lima Beans (large)	8-12 hrs.	45-60 min.	2
Lima Beans (small)	8-12 hrs.	50-60 min.	3
Mung Beans	-	60 min.	2
Navy Beans	6-8 hrs.	45-60 min.	2-2/3
Pink Beans	4-8 hrs.	50-60 min.	2-3/4
Pinto Beans	6-8 hrs.	1-1/2	2-2/3
Soybeans	8-12 hrs.	1-2 hrs.	3
Tepary Beans	8-12 hrs.	90 min.	3

*The recommended times in this chart are approximate.

A pressure cooker will reduce the amount of cooking time needed. A 15-pound pressure cooker will reduce cooking time by 600%. In other words, what would normally take 1 hour, takes only 10 minutes with a pressure cooker. Adding Kombu seaweed to an overnight soak also speeds up cooking time by about 200%.

To test whether your beans are ready to be eaten, remove one from the pot, allow it to cool and place it between your tongue and the roof of your mouth. Apply pressure with your tongue. If it 'smooshes' easily, the beans are ready.

SPROUTING

An alternative to soaking is sprouting. This means activating *germination* in a seed. It takes longer than soaking but makes the nutrients in the seed more available for absorption. The process effectively reduces the anti-nutrient phytate by 37-81% in various types of grains and legumes.

Start by rinsing the seeds and then place them in cold water for 2-12 hours. After soaking, rinse the seeds again. The soaked seeds should then go into a sprouter- after various lengths of time depending on the bean or seed. If you don't have a sprouter, a deep plate covered by a lid or towel works. Rinse the seeds every 8 to 12 hours. When the beans, grains or legumes have sprouted a root, they are ready to be cooked.

Below is a list of sprouting times for various nuts, beans, legumes, seeds and grains:

- Almond: 12 hours
- Adzuki beans: 3-5 days
- Chickpea: 12 hours
- Lentil: 12 hours
- Kamut: 2-3 days
- Wheat: 2-3 days
- Oats: 2-3 days
- Spelt & Rye: 2-3 days
- Barley: 2 days
- Buckwheat: 1-2 days
- Quinoa: 1-2 days
- Millet: 2-3 days

- Rice: 3-5 days
- Corn: 2-3 days
- Pepita: 1-2 days
- Fenugreek: 3-5 days
- Black beans: 3 days
- White beans: 2-3 days
- Mung beans: 2-5 days
- Kidney beans: 5-7 days
- Navy beans: 2-3 days
- Peas: 2-3 days
- Amaranth grains: 1-3 days
- Wheat berries: 3-4 days

- Wild rice: 3-5 days
- Black rice: 3-5 days
- Radish seeds: 3-4 days
- Alfalfa seeds: 3-5 days
- Pumpkin seeds: 1-2 days
- Sesame seeds: 1-2 days
- Sunflower seeds: 2-3 days

Soaking and sprouting chia, hemp and flaxseeds

Like with other seeds, soaking chia, hemp and flaxseeds maximizes nutrient availability and seed digestibility.

To soak chia seeds, place seeds in a jar or glass and add water. Shake it for 2-3 minutes and place the container in the fridge. To fully soak the seeds, refrigerate for at least 1 hour. An overnight soak is ideal in order to achieve the gel-like consistency of the mixture you are aiming for.

Tip: Use a mason jar so that seeds can be kept in the fridge for longer periods. Since this seed does not go bad easily, it is possible to always have some ready in the fridge.

Hemp seeds are one of the most easily digested plant protein sources and do not require soaking—they can be consumed dry.

Flaxseeds, on the other hand, are prepared in a similar way to chia seeds. Place them in a jar with water and shake before leaving them to soak for 10 minutes to 2 hours at room temperature. The water will turn opaque from the soluble fibers and gums. This water can be re-used to cook with and will contribute additional nutrients to a meal.

Sprouting

The process used to sprout smaller seeds like chia and flaxseed differs to that of larger seeds. These seeds have a mucilaginous coat which, when left in water, creates a gel-like mixture. Soak the seeds in a shallow dish and drain. Cover the dish with foil or move the seeds to a plastic bowl. Place the dish or bowl in a sunlit area and spray the seeds with water twice a day. After 3 to 7 days, the seeds will sprout.

Rice

Rice is a popular staple food and comes in many varieties. Each variety requires its own preparation method. Brown rice, for example, requires more water and takes longer to cook than white rice. Rice can be cooked in a rice cooker, pot or steamer.

TYPES OF RICE:

- Long-grain rice – fluffy grains that stay separated (basmati, jasmine, red cargo)
- Medium-grain rice – tender, moist and chewy (brown, rosematta)
- Short-grain rice – short and plump, stick together and clump up (sticky, sushi, Valencia)

It is a good idea to rinse rice prior to cooking. This is done to remove excess starch. Short-grain does not require rinsing as the starch provides the desired texture for the dishes in which short-grain rice is used.

COOKING IN A POT

METHOD FOR LONG-GRAIN RICE:

1. Measure the rice into a cup, level the top.
2. Rinse the rice with cold water until the water is clear.
3. Optional: soak the rice for up to 30 minutes and drain.
4. Pour the rinsed rice into a pot.
5. Add double the amount of water, 2 cups for 1 cup of dry rice.
6. Optional: add a pinch of salt and oil of choice.
7. Bring the water to a soft boil.
8. Put the lid on top of the pot and softly shake the pot to distribute the rice evenly.
9. Cook for 10 minutes with the lid on.
10. When all water is absorbed, turn off the heat, take off the lid and cover the pot with a tea towel.
11. Set aside for the recipe or serve and enjoy!

METHOD FOR MEDIUM-GRAIN RICE:

1. Measure the rice into a cup, level the top.
2. Rinse the rice in a strainer with cold water to improve texture and get rid of grit and dust.
3. Add 2 cups water for each cup of (brown) rice
4. Optional: add a little olive oil.
5. Bring the water to a boil, lower the heat and cook the rice for 45 minutes.
6. Check the rice – Majority of water should be gone, a little water left in the pot is fine.
7. Drain excess water if necessary.
8. After cooking, allow the rice to rest with the lid on for about 10 minutes.
9. Fluff the rice with a fork and transfer it to a dish.
10. Set aside for a dish or recipe or consume and enjoy!

METHOD FOR SHORT-GRAIN RICE:

1. Measure the rice into a cup, level the top.
2. Wash the rice with a small amount of cold water to get rid of surface dust.
3. Fill a pot with the amount of water equal to the amount of rice.
4. Soak the rice for 15 minutes up to 3 hours.
5. Cover the pot and bring the water to a boil.
6. When the water is boiling, turn the heat to low.
7. Allow the rice to simmer for about 15 minutes without removing the lid.
8. When all the water is absorbed, a hissing sound is heard.
9. Turn off the heat, allow the rice to stand covered with the lid for 10 to 20 minutes.
10. Remove the lid and set the rice aside or serve and enjoy!

Type of rice	Water needed
White, long grain	1 ¾ - 2 cups per 1 cup rice
White, medium grain	1 ½ cups per 1 cup rice
White, short grain	1 ¼ cups per 1 cup rice
Brown, long grain	2 ¼ cups per 1 cup rice
Brown, medium grain	2 cups per 1 cup rice

For drier rice (Basmati or Jasmin), use slightly less water than displayed above.

COOKING IN A RICE COOKER

A rice cooker is an automated device that adjusts cook time to different types of rice and keeps it warm after it is ready. Preparation steps are otherwise the same as described for the pot method.

Quinoa

Quinoa is common ingredient in many vegan recipes such as curry or salad recipes. This superfood is easy to cook and, like rice, comes in several different varieties such as white, red and black. White quinoa carries the most neutral flavor, while red and black have more distinct flavors and are often used in salads.

METHOD FOR PREPARING QUINOA:
1. Measure the quinoa into a cup, level the top.
2. Rinse the quinoa in a strainer with cold water thoroughly and drain.
3. Add 2 cups water for each cup of quinoa
4. Bring the water to a boil.
5. Optional: occasionally stir the quinoa with a wooden spoon.
6. Cover the pot with a lid.
7. Turn heat low and allow the quinoa to simmer for 15 minutes.
8. Take the pot off the heat and let the quinoa sit with the lid on top for 5 to 10 minutes.
9. Remove the lid, fluff and set aside or serve.
10. Enjoy!

ESSENTIAL RECIPES

1. Sweet Cashew Cheese Spread

Serves: 2 cups of cheese/10 servings | Prep Time: ~5 min |

Total number of ingredients: 3

Nutrition Information
(per serving)

- Calories: 153 kcal.
- Carbs: 7.8g.
- Fat: 11.4g.
- Protein: 4.8g.
- Fiber: 1.0g.
- Sugar: 1.7g.

INGREDIENTS:

- 5 drops stevia
- 2 cups raw cashews
- ½ cup water (optional)

METHOD:

1. Soak cashews for 6 hours in water.
2. Drain excess water and transfer the cashews to a food processor.
3. Add the stevia and optional water, depending on the desired thickness.
4. Blend until smooth.
5. For the best flavor, serve chilled.
6. Enjoy, use for another recipe or store!

STORAGE INFORMATION:

Storage	Temperature	Expiration date	Preparation
Airtight containerS	Fridge at 38 – 40°F or 3°C	4-5 days after preparation	
Airtight containerS	Freezer at -1°F or -20°C	60 days after preparation	Thaw at room temperature.

2. Flax Egg

Total number of ingredients: 2

Nutrition Information
(per serving)

- Calories: 37 kcal.
- Carbs: 2.1g.
- Fat: 2.7g.
- Protein: 1.1g.
- Fiber: 1.9g.
- Sugar: 0g.

INGREDIENTS:
- 1 tbsp. ground flaxseed
- 2-3 tbsp. lukewarm water

METHOD:
1. Mix the ground flaxseed with water in a cup.
2. Let the mixture sit, covered for 10 minutes.
3. Use the flax egg in a recipe or store.

STORAGE INFORMATION:

Storage	Temperature	Expiration date	Preparation
Airtight container S	Fridge at 38 – 40°F or 3°C	3-4 days after preparation	
Airtight container S	Freezer at -1°F or -20°C	60 days after preparation	Thaw at room temperature.

Note: You can use this mixture to replace a single egg in any recipe.

3. Mexican Salsa

Total number of ingredients: 6

Nutrition Information
(per serving)
- Calories: 30 kcal.
- Carbs: 6.1g.
- Fat: 0.3g.
- Protein: 0.8g.
- Fiber: 2.1g.
- Sugar: 4.2g.

INGREDIENTS:
- 4 firm tomatoes (large)
- 1 fresh jalapeno
- 2 tbsp. fresh cilantro (chopped)
- ½ red onion (medium, diced)
- 1 lime
- Salt and black pepper to taste

METHOD:
1. Skin and seed the tomatoes. Halve the jalapeno and remove the stem, seeds and placenta.
2. Cut the tomatoes and jalapeno into fine pieces.
3. Add the cut veggies to a medium size bowl.
4. Chop the cilantro and red onion into tiny bits and add to the bowl.
5. Juice the lime into the bowl and stir the ingredients well.
6. Season the mixture to taste with salt and black pepper.
7. After all the ingredients are combined, let it sit in the fridge for one hour before serving.
8. Enjoy, share or store for later!

STORAGE INFORMATION:

Storage	Temperature	Expiration date	Preparation
Airtight container S	Fridge at 38 – 40°F or 3°C	3-4 days after preparation	
Airtight container S	Freezer at -1°F or -20°C	60 days after preparation	Thaw at room temperature.

4. Apple Sauce

Serves: 4 | Prep Time: ~40 min |

Total number of ingredients: 6

Nutrition Information
(per serving)
- Calories: 202 kcal.
- Carbs: 50.5g.
- Fat: 0g.
- Protein: 0g.
- Fiber: 8.9g.
- Sugar: 38g.

INGREDIENTS:
- 4 Jazz apples (skinned, cored, cubed)
- 4 Red Delicious apples (skinned, cored, cubed)
- ½ cup water
- Pinch of salt
- ½ tsp. cinnamon (optional)
- 1 tbsp. lemon juice (optional)

METHOD:
1. Skin and core the apples, cut them into small cubes or quarters and put these in cold water for about 5 minutes.
2. Take the apple parts out and cut these into slices.
3. Add the ½ cup of water to a saucepan over medium heat and add a pinch of salt and the apple slices.
4. Make sure to stir often while slowly heating the mixture until it cooks.
5. After the boiling point has been reached, turn down the heat to low.
6. Mash the apples while simmering to create a sauce in about 10 minutes.
7. Keep stirring and mashing until you have a chunky applesauce. This should take about 20 minutes.
8. Add the optional cinnamon and lemon juice.
9. Let it cool. Blend in a blender or food processor for a smoother applesauce.
10. Serve chilled or store for later!

STORAGE INFORMATION:

Storage	Temperature	Expiration date	Preparation
Airtight containerS	Fridge at 38 – 40°F or 3°C	3-4 days after preparation	
Airtight containerS	Freezer at -1°F or -20°C	60 days after preparation	Thaw at room temperature.

5. Cashew Cheese Spread

**Serves: 1 cup of cheese /
5 servings | Prep Time: ~5 min |**

Total number of ingredients: 5

Nutrition Information
(per serving)
- Calories: 151kcal.
- Carbs: 8.8g.
- Fat: 10.9g.
- Protein: 4.6g.
- Fiber: 1.0g.
- Sugar: 1.7g.

INGREDIENTS:
- 1 cup water
- 1 cup raw cashews
- 1 tsp. nutritional yeast
- ½ tsp. salt
- 1 tsp. garlic powder (optional)

METHOD:
1. Soak the cashews for 6 hours in a medium-sized bowl filled with water.
2. Drain and transfer the soaked cashews to a food processor.
3. Add 1 cup water and all the other ingredients and blend.
4. For the best flavor, serve chilled.
5. Enjoy or store for later!

STORAGE INFORMATION:

Storage	Temperature	Expiration date	Preparation
Airtight container M	Fridge at 38 – 40°F or 3°C	4-5 days after preparation	
Airtight container M	Freezer at -1°F or -20°C	60 days after preparation	Thaw at room temperature.

6. Puffed Brown Rice

Serves: 4 servings/1 cup | Prep Time: ~15 min |

Total number of ingredients: 2

Nutrition Information
(per serving)
- Calories: 47 kcal.
- Carbs: 5.63g.
- Fat: 2.48g.
- Protein: 1.25g.
- Fiber: 0.6g.
- Sugar: 0g.

INGREDIENTS:
- ½ cup dry brown rice
- 4-8 cups of MCT oil

METHOD:

1. Line a medium bowl with paper towels. This is for absorbing the excess oil after puffing the rice.
2. Pour about 4-8 cups MCT oil in a medium sauce pan and heat over high heat; make sure that there is enough oil in the pan to cover an entire metal sieve.
3. Check if the oil is hot enough by throwing in a few grains. If these sizzle and puff up, the oil is hot enough.
4. Place the dry rice grains in the sieve and carefully lower it into the oil until it is fully covered. Shake gently to make sure everything puffs up. It will puff quickly so make sure to watch the process carefully. Avoid burning the rice.
5. Remove the sieve with puffed rice and transfer the puffed grains into the bowl.
6. Let it cool down and discard the excess oil.
7. Use the puffed rice for the desired recipe, enjoy or store!

STORAGE INFORMATION:

Storage	Temperature	Expiration date	Preparation
Airtight containers	Fridge at 38 – 40°F or 3°C	4-5 days after preparation	
Airtight containers	Freezer at -1°F or -20°C	60 days after preparation	Thaw at room temperature.

7. Chocolate Hazelnut Spread

Total number of ingredients: 6

Nutrition Information
(per serving)
- Calories: 239 kcal.
- Carbs: 7.1g.
- Fat: 20.6g.
- Protein: 6.4g.
- Fiber: 5.3g.
- Sugar: 2.6g.

INGREDIENTS:
- 2 cups raw hazelnuts (can be re-placed with cashews)
- ¼ cup coconut cream
- 1-2 tbsp. cocoa powder
- 1 tsp. stevia
- ½ tsp. vanilla extract
- ½ tsp. coffee beans, (grounded, optional)

METHOD:
1. Preheated the oven to 300°F or 150°C.
2. Roast the hazelnuts (or cashews) on a baking sheet lined with parchment paper.
3. After about 12 minutes, take out the nuts and let them cool down.
4. Put all the ingredients in blender or food processor.
5. Blend until smooth. Add more water if necessary. Stop and scrape down the edges of the blender or food processor if necessary.
6. Store, use for another recipe or enjoy!

STORAGE INFORMATION:

Storage	Temperature	Expiration date	Preparation
Airtight container M	Fridge at 38 – 40°F or 3°C	5 days after preparation	
Airtight container M	Freezer at -1°F or -20°C	60 days after preparation	Thaw at room temperature.

8. Vegan Half & Half Cream

Serves: 8 | Prep Time: ~60 min |

Total number of ingredients: 2

Nutrition Information
(per serving)
- Calories: 106 kcal.
- Carbs: 2.4g.
- Fat: 10.3g.
- Protein: 1.0g.
- Fiber: 0.7g.
- Sugar: 0.8g.

INGREDIENTS:
- ½ can full-fat coconut milk
- ½ cup coconut cream

METHOD:
1. Heat a small saucepan over low heat.
2. Pour the coconut milk in.
3. Cut up the coconut cream if necessary and add it the coconut milk.
4. Keep stirring until the cream is dissolved.
5. Use warm or cold.
6. Enjoy, refrigerate or freeze.

STORAGE INFORMATION:

Storage	Temperature	Expiration date	Preparation
Airtight container S	Fridge at 38 – 40°F or 3°C	3 days after preparation	
Airtight container S	Freezer at -1°F or -20°C	60 days after preparation	Thaw at room temperature.

9. Chili Garlic Paste

Total number of ingredients: 6

Nutrition Information
(per serving)
- Calories: 116 kcal.
- Carbs: 5.9g.
- Fat: 9.8g.
- Protein: 1.2g.
- Fiber: 2g.
- Sugar: 0.8g.

INGREDIENTS:
- ½ cup MCT oil
- 1 cup green chili flakes
- 2 heads of garlic (medium, minced)
- 1 tsp. salt
- 2 tsp. sugar (optional)
- ¼ cup Szechuan peppercorns (optional)

METHOD
1. Put all the ingredients into a blender or food processor and blend until smooth.
2. Store or use right away with another recipe or as a topping.

STORAGE INFORMATION

Storage	Temperature	Expiration date	Preparation
Airtight container S	Fridge at 38 – 40°F or 3°C	14 days after preparation	
Airtight container S	Freezer at -1°F or -20°C	60 days after preparation	Thaw at room temperature.

10. Pie Crust

Total number of ingredients: 4

Nutrition Information
(per serving)
- Calories: 1157 kcal.
- Carbs: 131g.
- Fat: 59.6g.
- Protein: 24.2g.
- Fiber: 19.7g.
- Sugar: 1.7g.

INGREDIENTS:

- 1½ cup whole wheat flour
- Pinch of sugar and salt
- ¼ cup coconut oil (melted)
- ¼ cup almond milk

METHOD:

1. For the fully cooked pie crust; preheat oven to 355°F or 180°C.
2. Combine the flour, salt and sugar in a large bowl and mix well.
3. Add coconut oil and mix with a spoon until the mixture becomes a crumbly dough.
4. Blend in almond milk and mix again until everything can be formed into a ball of dough.
5. Roll out the dough on a flat surface covered with a tea towel. Use some flour to prevent sticking. Roll the dough out to be a bit larger than a pie dish.
6. Use the towel to flip the dough into pie dish and press it down. Cut down excess edges to form a nice crust.
7. Store for later or bake the crust for about 18 minutes until lightly browned.

STORAGE INFORMATION:

Storage	Temperature	Expiration date	Preparation
Ziploc bag or wrapping foil.	Fridge at 38 – 40°F or 3°C	2-3 days after preparation	
Ziploc bag or wrapping foil.	Freezer at -1°F or -20°C	60 days after preparation	Thaw at room temperature.

Tip: Use almond, spelt or coconut flour as an alternative.

11. Vegan Mayo

Total number of Ingredients: 10

Nutrition Information
(per serving)
 - Calories: 344 kcal.
 - Carbs: 1.3g.
 - Fat: 37.5g.
 - Protein: 0g.
 - Fiber: 0.2g.
 - Sugar: 1.2g.

INGREDIENTS:

 - 1 cup MCT oil
 - ½ cup almond milk
 - 1 tsp. lemon juice
 - 1 tsp. agave nectar
 - 1 tsp. rice vinegar
 - ½ tsp. mustard (ground)
 - 1 tsp. onion powder (optional)
 - 1 tsp. chili powder (optional)
 - 1 tsp. paprika powder (optional)
 - 1 clove garlic (optional)

METHOD

1. Put the almond milk, agave nectar, rice vinegar, mustard and optional ingredients into a blender and blend.
2. Slowly add the MCT oil to the blender while blending to emulsify the oil and almond milk.
3. When the mixture starts to thicken, add the lemon juice.
4. Store in a sealable glass jar or an airtight container.

STORAGE INFORMATION:

Storage	Temperature	Expiration date	Preparation
Airtight container S	Fridge at 38 – 40°F or 3°C	7-8 days after preparation	
Airtight container S	Freezer at -1°F or -20°C	60 days after preparation	Thaw at room temperature.

12. No-Salt Cream Cheese

**Serves: 1 block/ 15 wedge slices |
Prep Time: ~25 minutes |**

Total number of Ingredients: 5

Nutrition Information
(per serving)
- Calories: 133 kcal.
- Carbs: 5.6g.
- Fat: 10.9g.
- Protein: 3g.
- Fiber: 0.6g.
- Sugar: 1.1g.

INGREDIENTS:
- 2 cups cashews
- ½ cup almond milk
- ¼ cup olive oil
- ½ tbsp. coconut vinegar
- 1 tsp. nutritional yeast

METHOD
1. Fill a medium pot with water and put it on the stove over medium heat.
2. Bring the water to a boil.
3. Continue to boil the cashews in the pot for up to 15 minutes.
4. Once cooked, strain the cashews and drain the excess water.
5. Place the cashews in a blender and blend until smooth.
6. Reuse the same pot and bring the almond milk, olive oil, nutritional yeast and vinegar to a simmer.
7. After 2 minutes, place the almond milk, olive oil and vinegar in a mixing bowl.
8. Slowly blend in the crushed cashews and stir the mixture into a smooth puree.
9. Mold into a block of cheese.
10. Enjoy or store!

STORAGE INFORMATION:

Storage	Temperature	Expiration date	Preparation
Airtight container M or Ziploc bag	Fridge at 38 – 40°F or 3°C	3-4 days after preparation	
Airtight container M or Ziploc bag	Freezer at -1°F or -20°C	60 days after preparation	Thaw at room temperature.

13. Vegetable Broth

Serves: 5 cups |
Prep Time: ~120 min |

Total number of ingredients: 15

Nutrition Information
(per serving)

- Calories: 0 kcal.
- Carbs: 0g.
- Fat: 0g.
- Protein: 0g.
- Fiber: 0g.
- Sugar: 0g.

INGREDIENTS:

- 10 cups water
- 2 onions (chopped)
- 3 cloves garlic (medium, minced)
- 4 carrots (chopped)
- 3 celery ribs (leafless, chopped)
- 1 sweet potato (cubed)
- 1 red bell pepper (sliced)
- 1 cup kale (fresh or frozen, cut)
- ½ cup parsley (fresh)
- ½ cup olive oil
- 1 tbsp. miso paste
- 2 tbsp. nutritional yeast (optional)
- 1 tbsp. thyme
- 1 tbsp. rosemary
- Salt and black pepper to taste

METHOD:

1. Preheat oven at 400°F or 200°C.
2. Toss the onions, garlic, carrots, celery, sweet potato, bell pepper, kale and parsley with the ½ cup of olive oil in an oven-proof roasting pan or baking tray.
3. Bake the veggies in the oven for about 20 minutes until browned and caramelized.
4. Put a large pot over medium heat and boil about 10 cups of water.
5. Add all ingredients from the roasting pan to the pot with boiling water.
6. Immediately bring the heat down to low and keep it at boiling point.
7. Stir every few minutes and add the miso paste, nutritional yeast, thyme and rosemary.
8. Add salt, pepper and any other desired spices to taste.
9. Cook until half of the water has evaporated.
10. Take the pot off the stove and let it cool.
11. Pour the mixture through a sieve and collect the broth in a second pot. Don't waste the veggies afterwards, it makes for a nice side dish.
12. Use or store!

STORAGE INFORMATION:

Storage	Temperature	Expiration date	Preparation
Airtight container L	Fridge at 38 – 40°F or 3°C	5 days after preparation	Reheat in microwave or pot
Airtight container L	Freezer at -1°F or -20°C	60 days after preparation	Thaw at room temperature. Reheat in microwave or pot

Tip: When freezing, divide the broth into smaller portions for convenient use.

14. Cream Cheese

Serves: 1 block / 15 wedge slices |
Prep Time: ~2 minutes |

Total number of Ingredients: 6

Nutrition Information
(per slice)
- Calories: 74 kcal.
- Carbs: 2.3g.
- Fat: 6.8g.
- Protein: 1.0g.
- Fiber: 0.4g.
- Sugar: 0g.

INGREDIENTS:
- ½ tsp. sea salt
- 1 tsp. non-dairy probiotic powder
- 1 tsp. nutritional yeast
- 2 cups organic coconut cream
  (chilled)
- 1 tsp. garlic powder
- Fresh herbs to taste (optional)

METHOD
1. Whisk the salt, probiotic powder, yeast and chilled coconut cream in a medium bowl until smooth.
2. Wrap the mixture in a cheese cloth or coffee filter in a container or the previously used bowl to cope with leaking and put it in the fridge for 24 hours.
3. After the 24 hours, unwrap the cheese mixture, add the salt and garlic powder and mix.
4. Cool the cheese in the fridge for another 6 hours.
5. Enjoy or store.

STORAGE INFORMATION:

Storage	Temperature	Expiration date	Preparation
Airtight container M	Fridge at 38 – 40°F or 3°C	3 days after preparation	
Airtight container M	Freezer at -1°F or -20°C	60 days after preparation	Thaw at room temperature.

15. Avocado Pesto

Serves: 2 cups/8 servings| Prep Time: ~35 minutes |

Total number of Ingredients: 9

Nutrition Information
(per serving)
 - Calories: 335 kcal.
 - Carbs: 4.7g.
 - Fat: 36.1g.
 - Protein: 1.0g.
 - Fiber: 3.7g.
 - Sugar: 0.4g.

INGREDIENTS:
 - 2 ripe avocadoes (peeled, pitted)
 - 1 cup extra virgin olive oil
 - 1 cup fresh spinach
 - ¼ cup fresh basil
 - 2 cloves garlic
 - 1 tsp. black pepper
 - 1 tbsp. oregano (fresh or dried)
 - 1 tbsp. rosemary (fresh or dried)
 - 1 tbsp. parsley (fresh or dried)

METHOD
1. Combine all the ingredients in a blender or food processor.
2. Blend thoroughly until smooth.
3. Serve and enjoy or store for later.

STORAGE INFORMATION:

Storage	Temperature	Expiration date	Preparation
Airtight container M	Fridge at 38 – 40°F or 3°C	1-2 days after preparation	
Airtight container M	Freezer at -1°F or -20°C	60 days after preparation	Thaw at room temperature.

16. Tortilla Wraps

Serves: 8 | Prep Time: ~15 minutes |

Total number of Ingredients: 4

Nutrition Information
(per serving)

- Calories: 81 kcal.
- Carbs: 11g.
- Fat: 4g.
- Protein: 2g.
- Fiber: 1.6g.
- Sugar: 0g.

INGREDIENTS:

- 2 ½ cups whole grain flour
- 2 tbsp. olive oil
- ½ cup water
- Pinch of salt

METHOD:

1. Pour 2 cups of flour into a bowl.
2. Add the olive oil, water and salt and mix well.
3. Add more water if the dough is too dry to mold and falls apart.
4. Make a big ball of dough and split into 8 equal parts.
5. Sprinkle a bit of flour on a flat surface for every ball.
6. Flatten the ball with your hands and sprinkle flour on the ball of dough when it gets too sticky.
7. Use a dough roller to flatten the ball into a thin circle. Spin the dough often to prevent it from sticking to the surface.
8. Make sure that your tortilla wrap is thin and about the size of a medium plate.
9. Put a large pan over high heat and cook the tortilla for about 30 seconds.
10. Repeat the process for the remaining balls to make 8 delicious tortillas.

STORAGE INFORMATION:

Storage	Temperature	Expiration date	Preparation
Ziploc bag or wrapping foil	Fridge at 38 – 40°F or 3°C	3-4 days after preparation	
Ziploc bag or wrapping foil	Freezer at -1°F or -20°C	60 days after preparation	Thaw at room temperature.

BREAKFAST RECIPES

1. Berry-Bana Smoothie Bag

Total number of Ingredients: 6

Nutrition Information
(per serving)
- Calories: 782 kcal.
- Carbs: 166g.
- Fat: 10g.
- Protein: 7g.
- Fiber: 37.8g.
- Sugar: 100g.

INGREDIENTS:
- 1 cup blueberries (fresh or frozen)
- 1 cup raspberries (fresh or frozen)
- 1 cup strawberries (fresh or frozen)
- 1 cup blackberries (fresh or frozen)
- 2 bananas (medium, sliced)
- 2 green apples (skinned, cored, cubed)
- 2 cups water

METHOD
1. Place all the ingredients except the water in a freezer-friendly Ziploc bag and then place this in the freezer.
2. When you are ready to make the smoothie, pour about 2 cups of water into the blender followed by the smoothie bag ingredients and blend well.
3. Serve and enjoy!

STORAGE INFORMATION:

Storage	Temperature	Expiration date	Preparation
Ziploc bag	Fridge at 38 – 40°F or 3°C	2-3 days after preparation	
Ziploc bag	Freezer at -1°F or -20°C	30 days after preparation	Thaw at room temperature.

2. Detox Smoothie Bowl

Total number of Ingredients: 10

Nutrition Information (per serving)

- Calories: 501 kcal.
- Carbs: 120.2g.
- Fat: 2.4g.
- Protein: 1.0g.
- Fiber: 22.9g.
- Sugar: 64g.

INGREDIENTS:

- 2 green apples (skinned, cored, chopped)
- 2 stalks celery (leafless)
- 1 cucumber (sliced)
- 2 ripe bananas (medium, sliced)
- ½ cup spinach
- ¼ cup fresh ginger root (chopped)
- 1 cup water

Toppings:

- ¼ cup blueberries (fresh or frozen)
- ¼ cup raspberries (fresh or frozen)
- 1 kiwi (skinned, sliced)

METHOD

1. Clean the spinach by rinsing and draining it with water if necessary.
2. Chop up the celery to fit in the blender.
3. Add all the ingredients except the toppings to blender.
4. Blend until smooth. Add water if necessary to reach the desired consistency.
5. Give it a good stir and pour into bowl.
6. Add toppings as you like and enjoy!

STORAGE INFORMATION:

Storage	Temperature	Expiration date	Preparation
2 compartment airtight container M/L	Fridge at 38 – 40°F or 3°C	2-3 days after preparation	
2 compartment airtight container M/L	Freezer at -1°F or -20°C	30 days after preparation	Thaw at room temperature.

Note: Store the ingredients unblended and keep the topping ingredients separated.

3. Garden Green Smoothie Bag

Serves: 1 | Prep Time: ~ 5 min |

Total number of Ingredients: 7

Nutrition Information
(per serving)
- Calories: 530 kcal.
- Carbs: 50.5g.
- Fat: 24g.
- Protein: 28g.
- Fiber: 37.5g.
- Sugar: 27g.

INGREDIENTS:
- 1 kiwi (peeled, halved)
- 1 cup spinach
- ½ cup kale
- 1 cup banana
- ½ cup flaxseeds (ground)
- ¼ cup chia seeds (optional)
- ¼ cup hemp seeds (optional)
- 1 ½ cups water

METHOD
1. Place all the ingredients except the water in a freezer-friendly Ziploc bag and then place this in the freezer.
2. When ready for use, pour about 1½ cups of water into the blender followed by the ingredients from the smoothie bag and blend well.
3. Serve and enjoy!

STORAGE INFORMATION:

Storage	Temperature	Expiration date	Preparation
Ziploc bag	Fridge at 38 – 40°F or 3°C	2-3 days after preparation	
Ziploc bag	Freezer at -1°F or -20°C	30 days after preparation	Thaw at room temperature.

4. Mango Blaster Smoothie Bag

Total number of Ingredients: 5

Nutrition Information
(per serving)
- Calories: 663 kcal.
- Carbs: 122g.
- Fat: 16.5g.
- Protein: 6.8g.
- Fiber: 22g.
- Sugar: 71g.

INGREDIENTS:
- 1 cup mango (chopped)
- 1 cup papaya (cubed)
- 1 cup blackberries (fresh or frozen)
- 2 bananas (medium, sliced)
- 1 cup coconut milk
- ½ cup water

METHOD
1. Place all the ingredients except the coconut milk and water, in a freezer-friendly Ziploc bag and place in the freezer.
2. When you are ready to make the smoothie, pour the coconut milk and ½ cup of water into the blender followed by the bag's ingredients and blend well.
3. Serve and enjoy!

STORAGE INFORMATION:

Storage	Temperature	Expiration date	Preparation
Ziploc bag	Fridge at 38 – 40°F or 3°C	2-3 days after preparation	
Ziploc bag	Freezer at -1°F or -20°C	30 days after preparation	Thaw at room temperature.

5. Energy Smoothie Bowl

Total number of Ingredients: 9

Nutrition Information
(per serving)

- Calories: 695 kcal.
- Carbs: 108.3g.
- Fat: 24.6g.
- Protein: 10.2g.
- Fiber: 15.5g.
- Sugar: 77.1g.

INGREDIENTS:

- 1 orange (skinned, parted)
- 2 frozen bananas (medium, chopped)
- ¼ cup fresh ginger root (sliced)
- ¼ cup fresh lemon juice
- ½ cup coconut milk
- ½ tsp. guarana (optional)

Toppings:

- ¼ cup walnuts
- ¼ cup goji berries (fresh or frozen)
- 1 kiwi (skinned, sliced)

METHOD

1. Add the orange, bananas, ginger, lemon juice, coconut milk and optional guarana to a blender.
2. Blend until smooth. Add water if necessary to reach the desired consistency.
3. Give it a good stir and pour into a bowl.
4. Add the toppings and enjoy!

STORAGE INFORMATION:

Storage	Temperature	Expiration date	Preparation
2 compartment airtight container M/L	Fridge at 38 – 40°F or 3°C	2-3 days after preparation	
2 compartment airtight container M/L	Freezer at -1°F or -20°C	30 days after preparation	Thaw at room temperature.

Note: Store the ingredients unblended and keep the topping ingredients separated.

6. Pineapple Sunrise Smoothie Bag

Total number of Ingredients: 5

Nutrition Information
(per serving)
- Calories: 543 kcal.
- Carbs: 120g.
- Fat: 4.5g.
- Protein: 5.8g.
- Fiber: 16g.
- Sugar: 86g.

INGREDIENTS:
- 1 cup pineapple
- 1 cup mango
- 1 cup blueberries (fresh or frozen)
- 1 banana sliced
- 1 orange (peeled, parted)
- 2 cups water

METHOD
1. Place all the ingredients except the water in a freezer-friendly Ziploc bag and then place this in the freezer.
2. When you are ready to make the smoothie, pour 2 cups of water into the blender followed by the smoothie bag ingredients and blend well.
3. Serve and enjoy!

STORAGE INFORMATION:

Storage	Temperature	Expiration date	Preparation
Ziploc bag	Fridge at 38 – 40°F or 3°C	2-3 days after preparation	
Ziploc bag	Freezer at -1°F or -20°C	30 days after preparation	Thaw at room temperature.

7. Berry Green Smoothie Bag

Serves: 1 | Prep Time: ~ 5 min |

Total number of Ingredients: 6

Nutrition Information
(per serving)
- Calories: 944 kcal.
- Carbs: 107g.
- Fat: 52g.
- Protein: 12g.
- Fiber: 18g.
- Sugar: 59.5g.

INGREDIENTS:
- 2 cups greens (i.e. spinach or kale, fresh or frozen)
- 3 cups mixed frozen berries (i.e. blueberries, strawberries, raspberries.)
- 1 banana (medium, sliced)
- ¼ cup walnuts (chopped)
- ¼ cup flax seeds (soaked, optional)
- ¼ cup hemp seeds (optional)
- 2 cups water

METHOD
1. Place all the ingredients except the water in a freezer-friendly Ziploc bag and then place this in the freezer.
2. When you are ready to make the smoothie, pour about 2 cups of water into the blender followed by the ingredients from the smoothie bag and blend well.
3. Serve and enjoy!

STORAGE INFORMATION:

Storage	Temperature	Expiration date	Preparation
Ziploc bag	Fridge at 38 – 40°F or 3°C	2-3 days after preparation	
Ziploc bag	Freezer at -1°F or -20°C	30 days after preparation	Thaw at room temperature.

8. Banana-Oat Cups

Serves: 6 | Prep Time: ~ 35 min |

Total number of Ingredients: 10

Nutrition Information
(per serving)
- Calories: 389 kcal.
- Carbs: 45g.
- Fat: 18g.
- Protein: 10.6g.
- Fiber: 15.5g.
- Sugar: 9.6g.

INGREDIENTS:
- 2½ cups old-fashioned rolled oats
- 3 cups water
- 1½ cups oat milk (unsweetened)
- 1 tbsp. coconut oil
- ½ cup flaxseeds (ground)
- ½ cup chia seeds
- 2 bananas (medium, sliced)
- 2-5 tsp. cinnamon powder (to taste)
- ¼ tsp. kosher salt (more or less to taste)
- 1 stick vanilla (crushed)

METHOD
1. Soak the chia seeds in a cup of water at room temperature.
2. Drain excess water after soaking the seeds for about 10-30 minutes.
3. Toast the rolled oats in a medium pot on medium heat.
4. Add the water, oat milk, coconut oil, flaxseeds and chia seeds to the toasted rolled oats.
5. Stir well and bring the mixture to a boil over medium low heat.
6. Once boiling, turn the stove down to low heat and, add in the bananas, cinnamon and a pinch of salt.
7. Stir the mixture well, while cooking slowly for about 10 minutes or until the desired consistency is reached.
8. Once the heat is turned off, add the vanilla extract and stir once more.
9. Take off the stove and let the mixture chill until cooled down.
10. Serve in a cup or pour into a mason jar for storage and enjoy!

STORAGE INFORMATION:

Storage	Temperature	Expiration date	Preparation
Airtight container or Mason Jar S/M	Fridge at 38 – 40°F or 3°C	4-5 days after preparation	
Airtight container or Mason Jar S/M	Freezer at -1°F or -20°C	60 days after preparation	Thaw at room temperature.

9. Peachy Mango Bowl

Total number of Ingredients: 9

Nutrition Information
(per serving)

- Calories: 903 kcal.
- Carbs: 99g.
- Fat: 49.5g.
- Protein: 15.4g.
- Fiber: 28.2g.
- Sugar: 68.6g.

INGREDIENTS:

- 1 peach (pitted, sliced)
- 1 mango (peeled, diced)
- 1 cup coconut milk
- 1 orange (skinned, parted)
- ¼ cup flaxseed (soaked)
- ½ cup pineapple chunks

Toppings:

- ¼ cup blueberries (fresh or frozen)
- ¼ cup pecans
- ¼ cup shredded coconut

METHOD

1. Add all the ingredients except the toppings to a blender.
2. Blend until smooth. Add water if necessary to reach the desired consistency.
3. Give it a good stir and pour the mixture into a bowl.
4. Add toppings as you like and enjoy!

STORAGE INFORMATION:

Storage	Temperature	Expiration date	Preparation
2 compartment airtight container M/L	Fridge at 38 – 40°F or 3°C	2-3 days after preparation	
2 compartment airtight container M/L	Freezer at -1°F or -20°C	30 days after preparation	Thaw at room temperature.

Note: Store the ingredients unblended and keep the topping ingredients separated.

10. Breakfast Oats Bowl

Serves: 1 | Prep Time: ~15 min |

Total number of Ingredients: 9

Nutrition Information
(per slice)

- Calories: 628 kcal.
- Carbs: 76.2g.
- Fat: 29.5g.
- Protein: 13.6g.
- Fiber: 14.1g.
- Sugar: 29.2g.

INGREDIENTS:

- 1 cup coconut milk
- ½ cup rolled oats
- 1 banana (medium, sliced)
- ¼ cup blueberries (fresh or frozen)
- ½ tsp. vanilla extract (optional)
- 1½ tsp. agave syrup (optional)

Toppings:

- ¼ cup walnuts
- ¼ cup raspberries (fresh or frozen)
- 1 tsp. chia seeds

METHOD

1. Combine the coconut milk, oats, banana and blueberries in a blender.
2. Add the optional vanilla and agave syrup.
3. Blend until smooth.
4. Pour into bowl.
5. Add the toppings and enjoy!

STORAGE INFORMATION:

Storage	Temperature	Expiration date	Preparation
2 compartment airtight container M/L	Fridge at 38 – 40°F or 3°C	2-3 days after preparation	
2 compartment airtight container M/L	Freezer at -1°F or -20°C	30 days after preparation	Thaw at room temperature.

Note: Store the ingredients unblended and keep the topping ingredients separated.

11. Protein Pancakes

Total number of Ingredients: 8

Nutrition Information
(per serving)
- Calories: 113 kcal.
- Carbs: 5.3g.
- Fat: 7.6g.
- Protein: 7.8g.
- Fiber: 3.8g.
- Sugar: 0.7g.

INGREDIENTS:
- 1 scoop vegan protein powder
- ¼ cup almond flour
- 1 tbsp. glucomannan powder
- 1½ cup water
- 1 tbsp. flaxseed oil
- 2 tbsp. olive oil
- 1 tsp. vanilla extract
- 1 tsp. baking powder

METHOD
1. Soak the glucomannan powder in ½ cup of water for a couple of minutes.
2. Combine the vegan protein powder, baking powder and almond flour in a medium bowl and set the dry ingredients aside.
3. Mix the vanilla extract and flaxseed oil with the soaked glucomannan.
4. Put a non-stick pan on the stove over medium heat and add two tablespoons olive oil.
5. Slowly stir the remaining cup of water into the dry flour mixture and combine thoroughly.
6. Add the glucomannan mixture and stir well.
7. Add a heap of batter to the pan and spread it out into a ¼ inch thick pancake.
8. Bake for 5 minutes on each side and repeat this for all the pancakes.
9. Enjoy or store!

STORAGE INFORMATION:

Storage	Temperature	Expiration date	Preparation
Ziploc bag	Fridge at 38 – 40°F or 3°C	3-4 days after preparation	Reheat in microwave.
Ziploc bag	Freezer at -1°F or -20°C	60 days after preparation	Thaw at room temperature. Reheat in microwave.

Note: Smaller pancakes are easier to store!

12. Matcha Morning Bowl

Serves: 1 | Prep Time: ~15 min |

Total number of Ingredients: 9

Nutrition Information
(per serving)
- Calories: 562 kcal.
- Carbs: 67.1g.
- Fat: 28g.
- Protein: 10.7g.
- Fiber: 15.9g.
- Sugar: 44.3g.

INGREDIENTS:

- 1 cup coconut milk
- 1 orange (skinned, parted)
- 1 cup kale (chopped)
- 1 banana (medium, sliced)
- ½ cup blueberries (fresh or frozen)
- 1 tsp. matcha powder

Toppings:
- ¼ cup pecans
- ¼ cup raspberries (fresh or frozen)
- 1 tsp. hemp seeds

METHOD

1. Combine the coconut milk, orange, kale, banana and blueberries in a blender.
2. Add the matcha powder.
3. Blend until smooth.
4. Pour the smoothie into a bowl.
5. Add toppings as you like and enjoy!

STORAGE INFORMATION:

Storage	Temperature	Expiration date	Preparation
2 compartment airtight container M/L	Fridge at 38 – 40°F or 3°C	2-3 days after preparation	
2 compartment airtight container M/L	Freezer at -1°F or -20°C	30 days after preparation	Thaw at room temperature.

Note: Store the ingredients unblended and keep the topping ingredients separated.

13. Early Morning Oat Bun

Serves: 8 slices | Prep Time: ~ 30 min |

Total number of Ingredients: 10

Nutrition Information
(per serving)
- Calories: 271 kcal.
- Carbs: 30g.
- Fat: 12.7g.
- Protein: 9.4g.
- Fiber: 6.8g.
- Sugar: 7.5g.

INGREDIENTS:

- ½ cup flaxseeds (soaked)
- 4 cups oatmeal
- 4 bananas (medium, ripe)
- 3 ½ cups almond milk (unsweetened)
- 1 ½ cup of water
- ½ cup hemp seeds
- 1 stick vanilla (crushed)
- 1 pinch of cinnamon
- ½ tsp. of stevia
- Kosher salt to taste

METHOD

1. Rinse and soak the flaxseeds according to the method. Drain off excess water.
2. Rinse the oatmeal before starting.
3. Mash the bananas and mix them in a bowl with the rinsed oatmeal and crushed vanilla.
4. Divide the mixture in two and put each half into large freezer-friendly Ziploc bags.
5. Place the bags in the freezer for 15 minutes.
6. Take the bags out the freezer, place the contents of the bag along with the almond milk, hemp seeds, flax seeds, cinnamon and stevia into a large pot and mix well.
7. Bring 1½ cups of water to a boil over medium heat.
8. Add the first mixture and cook it for about 3-5 minutes until the oats are soft. Take the oat mixture from the heat and allow it to cool down for about 5-10 minutes.
9. Line a bread tray with a sheet of baking paper and fill it about halfway with the oat mixture.
10. Place the tray in the fridge and cool the mixture for about 8 hours.
11. Take out the bread tray from the fridge and cut the bun into 8 slices.
12. Enjoy or store!

STORAGE INFORMATION:

Storage	Temperature	Expiration date	Preparation
Ziploc bag	Fridge at 38 – 40°F or 3°C	3-4 days after preparation	
Ziploc bag	Freezer at -1°F or -20°C	60 days after preparation	Thaw at room temperature.

LUNCH RECIPES

1. Chickpea Couscous

Serves: 6 | Prep Time: ~15 min |

Total number of Ingredients: 16

Nutrition Information
(per serving)

- Calories: 270 kcal.
- Carbs: 44.2g.
- Fat: 6g.
- Protein: 10g.
- Fiber: 12.4g.
- Sugar: 9g.

INGREDIENTS:

- 1 cup dry quinoa
- 2 cups of dry chickpeas
- 2 tbsp. extra virgin olive oil
- 1 onion (large, chopped)
- 1 red bell pepper (diced)
- 3 cloves garlic (minced)
- 2 tsp. ground cumin
- 2 tsp. ground coriander
- ½ tsp. ground turmeric
- 1 tsp. cayenne pepper
- 2 cups vegetable broth (page 63)
- 1 lb. sweet potatoes (peeled, cubed)
- 3 carrots (chopped)
- 1 tbsp. lemon juice
- Salt to taste
- 2 tbsp. cilantro (chopped)

METHOD

1. Prepare the quinoa according to the recipe.
2. Prepare the chickpeas according to the recipe.
3. Take a big skillet and put it on medium heat.
4. Add the olive oil.
5. Sauté the onions and red pepper and stir until browned.
6. Add the garlic, cumin, coriander, turmeric and cayenne pepper to the skillet and stir.
7. Continue to add the vegetable stock, potatoes and carrots.
8. Bring the mixture to a boil, turn the heat down and softly cook the mixture on low heat for 30-40 minutes, covered.
9. Add in the cooked chickpeas, stir and cook for another 3 minutes.
10. Turn off the heat and set the skillet aside.
11. Divide the cooked quinoa into the desired number of portions. Pour the veggie mixture, lemon juice and optionally some extra olive oil on top of the quinoa.
12. Add salt to taste and top the meal off with some cilantro before serving.
13. Enjoy or store the veggie mix and quinoa separately!

STORAGE INFORMATION:

Storage	Temperature	Expiration date	Preparation
2 compartment airtight container M/L	Fridge at 38 – 40°F or 3°C	2-3 days after preparation	Reheat in pot or microwave.
2 compartment airtight container M/L	Freezer at -1°F or -20°C	30 days after preparation	Thaw at room temperature. Reheat in pot or microwave.

Note: Alternatively, use separate containers to store the couscous and veggie mixture.

2. Black Bean Burgers

Serves: 8 | Prep Time: ~20 min |

Total number of Ingredients: 13

Nutrition Information
(per serving)
- Calories: 212 kcal.
- Carbs: 36.2g.
- Fat: 3.2g.
- Protein: 9.9 g.
- Fiber: 8.1g.
- Sugar: 3.5g.

INGREDIENTS:
- 4 cups dry black beans (rinsed, drained)
- 2 tbsp. olive oil
- 2 tbsp. garlic powder (or fresh, minced)
- ¾ cup sweet onion (chopped)
- ½ cup green bell pepper (minced)
- 2 tbsp. whole wheat flour
- 2 tbsp. warm water
- 1 tbsp. chili-garlic paste (page 57)
- 2 tsp. smoked paprika powder
- 2 tsp. cumin
- Salt and pepper to taste
- 4 slices brown bread (crumbled, ensure it is vegan-friendly)
- 1 cup flour (optional, as needed)

METHOD
1. Preheat oven to 350°F or 175°C.
2. Prepare the black beans according to the recipe.
3. Lightly grease a baking tray with olive oil.
4. Mash the black beans in a bowl and mix in the onions, bell peppers and garlic.
5. In a separate bowl, mix the flour, warm water, chili-garlic paste, paprika powder, cumin, and salt and pepper to taste well.
6. Stir the flour mixture into the black bean mix, add in the bread crumbs and knead until a sticky batter is formed.
7. Form the batter into burger patties. Use additional flour to dip both sides of each burger.
8. Put the patties on the baking tray.
9. Place the tray in the oven. Cook the burgers for about 10 minutes on each side until the middle is cooked and both outsides crispy.
10. Serve or store!

STORAGE INFORMATION:

Storage	Temperature	Expiration date	Preparation
Ziploc bag M/L	Fridge at 38 – 40°F or 3°C	3-4 days after preparation	Reheat in microwave.
Ziploc bag M/L	Freezer at -1°F or -20°C	60 days after preparation	Thaw at room temperature. Reheat in microwave.

3. Sweet Potato Chickpea Mingle

Serves: 2 | Prep Time: ~30 min |

Total number of Ingredients: 11

Nutrition Information
(per serving)
- Calories: 379 kcal.
- Carbs: 33.4g.
- Fat: 20.2g.
- Protein 16g.
- Fiber: 27.8g.
- Sugar: 8.4g.

INGREDIENTS:
- 1 cup dry chickpeas
- 1 sweet potato (large, cubed)
- ½ tsp. ground cumin
- 1 tbsp. fresh ginger (minced)
- 1 tsp. spicy paprika powder
- Salt and pepper to taste
- 2 tbsp. water
- 2 tbsp. coconut oil
- 1 garlic clove (minced)
- 5 tbsp. baba ganoush (page 98)
- 1 tsp. tabasco sauce

METHOD
1. Preheat oven to 400°F or 200°C.
2. Prepare the chickpeas according to the recipe.
3. Take a baking sheet and grease it with 1 tablespoon of coconut oil.
4. Roast the sweet potato cubes in the oven for about 20 minutes and check them every five minutes. Use a fork to see if the cubes are softened. Turn the potato cubes to roast evenly. Set aside after roasting.
5. Place the cumin, fresh ginger, paprika powder, salt, pepper and water in a medium-sized bowl.
6. Stir well and add more spices to taste.
7. Take a large skillet and grease it with 1 tablespoon of coconut oil.
8. Put it on low heat and add the cooked chickpeas along with the minced garlic.
9. Carefully mash the mixture with a fork.
10. Cook for 4 minutes and add salt and pepper to taste.
11. Combine the mixture with the baba ganoush and spice mixture.
12. Stir well.
13. Top the mixture with tabasco sauce and enjoy!
14. Serve the chickpea mingled with the roasted potatoes
15. Enjoy or store the ingredients separately.

STORAGE INFORMATION:

Storage	Temperature	Expiration date	Preparation
2 compartment airtight container M/L	Fridge at 38 – 40°F or 3°C	4-5 days after preparation	Reheat in pot or microwave.
2 compartment airtight container M/L	Freezer at -1°F or -20°C	30 days after preparation	Thaw at room temperature. Reheat in pot or microwave.

Tip: Serve the dish with extra baba ganoush on the side. Use multiple compartment or separate containers to store the potatoes and chickpea mingle.

4. Risotto

Total number of Ingredients: 11

Nutrition Information
(per serving)
- Calories: 406 kcal.
- Carbs: 43.6g.
- Fat: 22.1g.
- Protein: 8.3g.
- Fiber: 3.9g.
- Sugar: 5.9g.

INGREDIENTS:
- 1 cup dry brown rice
- 1 tbsp. of olive oil
- 1 large onion (diced)
- 4 garlic cloves (minced)
- ½ cup pumpkin (fresh or canned)
- 3 cups vegetable broth (page 63)
- ¼ tsp. dried thyme
- 1 whole bay leaf
- 4 ounces of mushrooms (chopped)
- Salt and pepper to taste
- ¼ cup cashew cheese spread (page 52)

METHOD
1. Cook the rice according to the recipe.
2. Heat a large skillet on medium heat and add the olive oil.
3. Sauté the onions until brown and stir in the minced garlic.
4. Add the pumpkin, 1 cup of the vegetable stock, thyme, bay leaf, salt, pepper and mushrooms.
5. Stir the mixture until all the liquid has been absorbed and add another cup of the vegetable broth.
6. Repeat the stirring process until it all the liquid has been absorbed and add the last cup of vegetable broth.
7. Stir in the rice until the risotto has thickened.
8. Top the risotto with the cashew cheese.
9. Turn down the heat and add the coconut milk.
10. Stir, serve and enjoy!

STORAGE INFORMATION:

Storage	Temperature	Expiration date	Preparation
Airtight container M/L	Fridge at 38 – 40°F or 3°C	4-5 days after preparation	Reheat in pot or microwave
Airtight container M/L	Freezer at -1°F or -20°C	60 days after preparation	Thaw at room temperature. Reheat in pot or microwave

5. Black Bean Soup

Serves: 4 | Prep Time: ~25 min |

Total number of Ingredients: 13

Nutrition Information
(per serving)
- Calories: 235 kcal.
- Carbs: 29g.
- Fat: 8.9g.
- Protein: 9.7g.
- Fiber: 7.9g.
- Sugar: 3g.

INGREDIENTS:
- 2 cups dry black beans
- 2 cups water
- 2 tbsp. olive oil
- ¼ cup green onions (chopped)
- ¼ cup white onions (chopped)
- ½ cup chopped mushrooms
- 4 garlic cloves (chopped)
- ½ cup red bell peppers (chopped)
- 2 tsp. chili powder
- 2 tsp. cumin
- 2 tsp. tabasco sauce
- Salt to taste
- Handful fresh parsley (optional, chopped)

METHOD
1. Prepare the black beans according to the recipe.
2. Transfer the cooked beans to a food processor or blender and add 1 cup of water.
3. Blend until the mixture is firm and smooth. Add more water if needed.
4. Put a medium-sized skillet on medium heat.
5. Add the olive oil, onions, mushrooms, garlic and red bell pepper.
6. Heat the vegetables for about 5 minutes and add the bean mixture with 1 cup of water.
7. Add more water, depending on the desired thickness.
8. Stir in the salt, chili powder, cumin and tabasco.
9. Turn the heat down to low and allow the soup to softly cook for 15 minutes, covered.
10. Serve with the optional fresh parsley on top.
11. Enjoy or store!

STORAGE INFORMATION:

Storage	Temperature	Expiration date	Preparation
Airtight container M/L	Fridge at 38 – 40°F or 3°C	4-5 days after preparation	Reheat in pot or microwave
Airtight container M/L	Freezer at -1°F or -20°C	60 days after preparation	Thaw at room temperature. Reheat in pot or microwave

6. Coconut Curry Lentil Soup

Serves: 2 | Prep Time: ~15 min |

Total number of Ingredients: 14

Nutrition Information
(per serving)
- Calories: 935kcal.
- Carbs: 90.7g.
- Fat: 51g.
- Protein: 29g.
- Fiber: 21.8g.
- Sugar: 17.8g.

INGREDIENTS:
- 2 cups dry red lentils
- 2 tbsp. coconut oil
- 3 onions, (medium, chopped)
- 3 garlic cloves (minced)
- ¼ cup fresh ginger (minced)
- 2 tbsp. tomato paste
- 2 tbsp. curry powder
- ½ tsp. hot red pepper flakes
- 4 cups vegetable broth (page 63)
- 1 jar diced tomatoes
- 1 can full-fat coconut milk
- 3 handfuls spinach (chopped)
- Salt and pepper to taste
- ¼ cup cilantro (chopped)

METHOD
1. Prepare the lentils according to the recipe.
2. Heat the coconut oil in a medium-sized stir-fry pan over medium heat.
3. Stir-fry the onion, garlic and ginger until these ingredients are translucent.
4. Add the tomato paste, curry powder and red pepper flakes.
5. Continue to add the vegetable broth, diced tomatoes and lentils.
6. Cover the pan and bring the mixture to a boil.
7. Add the lentils and coconut milk, turn the heat down to low and let the mixture slowly cook for about 15-20 minutes, covered.
8. Add salt and pepper to taste.
9. Stir in the chopped spinach.
10. Garnish with cilantro.
11. Enjoy warm or allow the soup to cool down before storage!

STORAGE INFORMATION:

Storage	Temperature	Expiration date	Preparation
Airtight container M/L	Fridge at 38 – 40°F or 3°C	4-5 days after preparation	Reheat in pot or microwave.
Airtight container M/L	Freezer at -1°F or -20°C	60 days after preparation	Thaw at room temperature. Reheat in pot or microwave.

Tip: Serve this dish with a small portion of long-grain or jasmine rice for extra carbs and fiber.

7. Spicy Black Bean Soup & Tortilla Chips

Serves: 3 | Prep Time: ~15 min |

Total number of Ingredients: 14

Nutrition Information
(per serving)
- Calories: 829 kcal.
- Carbs: 110g.
- Fat: 34g.
- Protein: 20.8g.
- Fiber: 16.8g.
- Sugar: 13g.

INGREDIENTS:
- 1 bag (300g) tortilla chips
- 2 cups dry black beans
- 2 tbsp. olive oil
- 2 yellow onions (large, chopped)
- 3 celery ribs (finely chopped)
- 2 carrots (medium, peeled and sliced)
- 4 cups vegetable broth (page 63)
- 6 garlic cloves (minced)
- 2 tbsp. ground cumin
- ½ tsp. red pepper flakes
- 3 tbsp. fresh lime juice
- 1 tsp. of sherry vinegar
- Sea salt and ground black pepper to taste
- 2 tsp. of lime juice

METHOD
1. Prepare the black beans according to the recipe.
2. Place a large soup pot on medium heat.
3. Add the olive oil, onions, celery and carrots to the pot.
4. Add a pinch of salt and blend in the vegetable broth.
5. Stir occasionally and cook the soup for about 10 minutes.
6. Add the garlic, cumin and pepper flakes.
7. Add the beans to the soup.
8. Lower the heat and let the soup simmer for about 20 minutes, covered.
9. Blend the soup in a blender until smooth (depending on the size of the blender, in 2-3 parts).
10. Return the blended soup to the soup pot.
11. Stir in the lime juice, sherry vinegar and pepper.
12. Add more spices like salt and pepper to taste.
13. Serve in a bowl with 100 g of tortilla chips on the side.
14. Enjoy or store!

STORAGE INFORMATION:

Storage	Temperature	Expiration date	Preparation
Airtight container M/L & Ziploc bag S	Fridge at 38 – 40°F or 3°C	4-5 days after preparation	Reheat the soup in pot or microwave
Airtight container M/L & Ziploc bag S	Freezer at -1°F or -20°C	60 days after preparation	Thaw at room temperature. Reheat the soup in pot or microwave

Note: Store the tortilla chips in separate Ziploc bags per portion to prevent deviant portion sizes. Alternatively keep the chips in the original package.

8. Mushroom Ragout

Total number of Ingredients: 10

Nutrition Information
(per serving)
- Calories: 77 kcal.
- Carbs: 4.2g.
- Fat: 4.1g.
- Protein: 2.5g.
- Fiber: 1.6g.
- Sugar: 2.2g.

INGREDIENTS:

- 2 tbsp. olive oil
- 1 sweet onion (big, finely chopped)
- 1 clove garlic (minced)
- 6 cups Portobello mushrooms (chopped)
- ½ cup dry red wine
- 1 cup vegetable broth (page 63)
- ½ tbsp. nutritional yeast
- ¼ cup basil leaves (chopped)
- ¼ cup no-salt cream cheese (page 61)
- ¼ cup parsley (optional, chopped)
- Salt and pepper to taste

METHOD

1. Take a large pot and put it on medium heat.
2. Sauté the onions and garlic in the olive oil while stirring.
3. Add some salt and pepper to taste and stir.
4. Mix in the mushrooms and turn up the heat a bit.
5. Cook and stir the mushrooms until most of the liquid in it has evaporated.
6. Add the red wine. Turn the heat up to medium-high and cook the ragout until most of the wine is evaporated.
7. Add the vegetable broth and stir thoroughly.
8. Blend in the nutritional yeast and cook the ragout for about 5 minutes.
9. Add the chopped basil and the no-salt cream cheese.
10. Lower the heat and keep stirring until the ragout simmers.
11. Keep stirring occasionally for about 5 more minutes and add more salt and pepper to taste.
12. Turn the heat off and set aside for about minutes to let the ragout cool down a bit.
13. Garnish with the optional parsley before serving and enjoy while warm or store.

STORAGE INFORMATION:

Storage	Temperature	Expiration date	Preparation
Airtight container M/L	Fridge at 38 – 40°F or 3°C	2-3 days after preparation	Reheat in pot or microwave
Airtight container M/L	Freezer at -1°F or -20°C	60 days after preparation	Thaw at room temperature. Reheat in pot or microwave

Tip: add in tofu or tempeh with the red wine to add extra protein to the recipe and serve with bread for dipping!

9. Easy Baba Ganoush

Serves: 2 | Prep Time: ~15 min |

Total number of Ingredients: 9

Nutrition Information
(per serving)
- Calories: 246 kcal.
- Carbs: 21.5g.
- Fat: 15.4g.
- Protein: 5.3g.
- Fiber: 8.3g.
- Sugar: 10.3g.

INGREDIENTS:
- 1 eggplant (large, sliced)
- 1 tbsp. MCT oil
- 4 tbsp. lemon juice
- 2 tbsp. tahini
- 2 garlic cloves (medium, minced)
- Salt and pepper to taste
- 2 tsp. sesame seeds (optional)
- Small carrot (optional, cut)
- Handful fresh cilantro, parsley or basil (optional, chopped)

METHOD
1. Preheat oven to 400°F or 200°C.
2. Put the sliced eggplant on a baking sheet.
3. Drizzle both sides of the eggplant with the MCT oil.
4. Put the baking sheet on a rack in the oven.
5. Allow the eggplant slices to broil for 2 minutes on each side.
6. Take the tray out of the oven and sprinkle the eggplant slices with salt.
7. Cover the tray with aluminum foil and put it back into the oven and allow the slices to steam for about 4 minutes.
8. Unwrap the eggplant, peel off its skin and transfer the eggplant to a blender.
9. Add the lemon juice, tahini, garlic, salt and pepper to taste and blend until smooth.
10. Transfer the mixture to a medium size bowl.
11. Top the baba ganoush with two or three of the optional ingredients.
12. Enjoy or store!

STORAGE INFORMATION:

Storage	Temperature	Expiration date	Preparation
Airtight container M/L	Fridge at 38 – 40°F or 3°C	3 days after preparation	
Airtight container M/L	Freezer at -1°F or -20°C	60 days after preparation	Thaw at room temperature.

Tip: Serve the baba ganoush with some fresh pita bread or grilled sweet potatoes!

10. Pumpkin Pilaf

Serves: 2 | Prep Time: ~20 min |

Total number of Ingredients: 13

Nutrition Information
(per serving)
- Calories: 557 kcal.
- Carbs: 90.1g.
- Fat: 16,8g.
- Protein: 11.5g.
- Fiber: 12.5g.
- Sugar: 13.1g.

INGREDIENTS:
- 2 cups dry brown rice
- 2 tbsp. olive oil
- 1 sweet potato (medium, cubed)
- 2 cups fresh pumpkin (cubed)
- 2 cups kale (fresh or frozen)
- 2 celery ribs (medium, cut)
- 1 onion (medium, cut)
- 2 garlic cloves
- 1 tbsp. onion powder
- 1 bay leaf (chopped)
- Salt and black pepper to taste
- ½ cup pumpkin seeds (optional)
- Handful of fresh parsley (chopped, optional)

METHOD
1. Cook the rice according to the recipe.
2. Put a large skillet on medium heat and add the olive oil to the skillet.
3. Throw in the sweet potato and pumpkin cubes.
4. Add the kale, onion, celery, garlic and onion powder.
5. Cook the mixture for 15-20 minutes and turn the heat down to low.
6. Add the cooked rice, optional pumpkin seeds, a handful of fresh parsley and stir thoroughly.
7. Softly cook the mixture for another 5 minutes.
8. Enjoy or store the pilaf for another day!

STORAGE INFORMATION:

Storage	Temperature	Expiration date	Preparation
Airtight container M/L	Fridge at 38 – 40°F or 3°C	2-3 days after preparation	Reheat in pot or microwave
Airtight container M/L	Freezer at -1°F or -20°C	60 days after preparation	Thaw at room temperature. Reheat in pot or microwave

11. Watermelon Soy Bowl

Serves: 2 | Prep Time: ~15 min |

Total number of Ingredients: 13

Nutrition Information
(per serving)
- Calories: 525 kcal.
- Carbs: 58.5g.
- Fat: 27g.
- Protein: 12g.
- Fiber: 13.4g.
- Sugar: 17.3g.

INGREDIENTS:

Watermelon mixture:
- 2 cups watermelon (cut, cubed)
- 4 tbsp. soy sauce
- 2 tbsp. sesame oil
- 2 yellow onions (medium, chopped)
- ½ tsp. rice vinegar
- ½ tsp. agave nectar
- 1 tsp. red pepper flakes
- Roasted sesame seeds to taste (optional)

Bowl contents:
- 1 cup brown rice
- 1 cucumber (sliced)
- 2 carrots (medium, sliced)
- 1 avocado (mashed)
- Wasabi avocado paste (optional; page 124, spicy beet bowl recipe)

METHOD

1. Cook the rice according to the recipe.
2. Add the watermelon cubes to a large bowl.
3. Blend in the soy sauce, sesame oil, yellow onion, agave nectar, rice vinegar and red pepper flakes.
4. Top the mixture with the optional roasted sesame seeds.
5. Cover the bowl and set it in the fridge for 3 hours.
6. Serve the rice in a medium bowl with the sliced cucumber, carrot and mashed avocado.
7. Top the rice with the optional wasabi avocado paste.
8. Take the watermelon mixture from the fridge and serve a big scoop on top of the rice mixture.
9. Enjoy or store!

STORAGE INFORMATION:

Storage	Temperature	Expiration date	Preparation
3-compartment airtight container M/L	Fridge at 38 – 40°F or 3°C	2-3 days after preparation	
3-compartment airtight container M/L	Freezer at -1°F or -20°C	60 days after preparation	Thaw at room temperature.

Note: Store the rice, vegetables and watermelon mixture in a multiple compartment container or separate containers.

12. Black Bean and Quinoa Burrito

Serves: 6 | Prep Time: ~20 min |

Total number of Ingredients: 17

Nutrition Information
(per serving)

- Calories: 493 kcal.
- Carbs: 84g.
- Fat: 8.8g.
- Protein: 16.5g.
- Fiber: 14.5g.
- Sugar: 6.6g.

INGREDIENTS:

- 2 cups dry black beans
- ½ cup dry quinoa
- 2 tbsp. canola oil
- 2 onions (medium, diced)
- 5 cloves garlic (minced)
- 1 jalapeño (seeded, minced)
- 1 red bell pepper (large, diced)
- 1 zucchini (medium, diced)
- 1 (200g) can of sweet corn (drained)
- 1 large tomato (diced)
- 1 tbsp. cumin
- 1 tsp. sweet paprika powder
- 1 tsp. chili powder
- 1 tsp. salt
- ½ bunch of cilantro (chopped)
- 2 tsp. lemon juice
- 6 tortillas (large, whole wheat)

METHOD

1. Prepare the black beans according to the recipe.
2. Prepare the quinoa according to the recipe.
3. Grease a large skillet with canola oil and put it on medium heat.
4. Sauté the onions for about 5 minutes until browned.
5. Add the garlic and jalapeños to the skillet and stir the ingredients for about 2 minutes.
6. Toss in the zucchini, jalapeño, red bell pepper, corn and tomato.
7. Cook the mixture for about 5 minutes while stirring.
8. Stir in the cooked beans, cumin, paprika powder, chili powder and add salt to the mix.
9. Add the cooked quinoa to the skillet. Stir everything before removing the skillet from the heat.
10. Put 4-5 tablespoons of the mixture on a tortilla and top it with fresh cilantro and lemon juice.
11. Wrap it tightly and enjoy right away or store the mixture and tortillas separately!

STORAGE INFORMATION:

Storage	Temperature	Expiration date	Preparation
Airtight container M/L and Ziploc bag	Fridge at 38 – 40°F or 3°C	3-4 days after preparation	Reheat in pot or microwave
Airtight container M/L and Ziploc bag	Freezer at -1°F or -20°C	60 days after preparation	Thaw at room temperature. Reheat in pot or microwave

Note: Use a container and a Ziploc bag for the tortillas and black bean mixture. Keep the cilantro in the original package and take out a small portion on the day of consumption. Same goes for the lemon; alternatively, slice a lemon in 3-6 pieces and wrap these in foil.

13. Sweet Potato Curry Soup

Serves: 3 | Prep Time: ~10 min |

Total number of Ingredients: 10

Nutrition Information
(per serving)
- Calories: 376 kcal.
- Carbs: 56.5g.
- Fat: 14 g.
- Protein: 5g.
- Fiber: 11g.
- Sugar: 15.6g.

INGREDIENTS:

- 1 tbsp. olive oil
- 2 brown onions (medium, chopped)
- 4 cloves garlic (minced)
- 5g. fresh ginger (sliced)
- 2 (14oz) cans unsweetened coconut milk
- 3 sweet potatoes (large, peeled, cubed)
- 1 can green chilies (diced)
- 2 tbsp. curry powder
- ½ tsp. cumin
- Salt and pepper to taste

METHOD

1. Take a large pot, put it over medium heat and add the olive oil.
2. Add the onions and stir until the onions start to brown.
3. Stir in the garlic, add the ginger and let it cook for a minute while stirring.
4. Pour in the coconut milk and then add all the remaining ingredients.
5. Cook over medium-low heat for about 45 minutes or until the potatoes reach the desired softness.
6. Mash or process the soup in a blender until the desired consistency or for about 2 minutes.
7. Serve the soup with salt, black pepper and add additional spices like ginger, curry or chili powder to taste.
8. Enjoy warm or allow the soup to cool down for storage!

STORAGE INFORMATION:

Storage	Temperature	Expiration date	Preparation
Airtight container M/L	Fridge at 38 – 40°F or 3°C	3-4 days after preparation	Reheat in pot or microwave
Airtight container M/L	Freezer at -1°F or -20°C	60 days after preparation	Thaw at room temperature. Reheat in pot or microwave

14. BBQ Bean Bowl

Serves: 3 | Prep Time: ~15 min |

Total number of Ingredients: 13

Nutrition Information
(per serving)
- Calories: 215 kcal.
- Carbs: 25g.
- Fat: 10g.
- Protein: 6g.
- Fiber: 21g.
- Sugar: 5g.

INGREDIENTS:
- 1 cup dry black beans
- ½ cup raw quinoa
- 2 tbsp. olive oil
- 1 zucchini (large, chopped)
- 1 red bell pepper (seeded, chopped)
- 1 green bell pepper (seeded, chopped)
- ½ red onion (chopped)
- Salt and pepper to taste

BBQ Vinaigrette:
- 2 tbsp. white wine vinegar
- 3 tbsp. BBQ sauce (vegan)
- 2 tsp. fresh lime juice
- ½ tsp. chili powder
- ½ tsp. salt

METHOD
1. Prepare the black beans according to the recipe.
2. Prepare the quinoa according to the recipe.
3. Put the olive oil into a large skillet.
4. Toss in the zucchini, bell peppers and onions.
5. Add the salt and black pepper to taste and stir well.
6. Transfer the mixture to a grill top or stove on medium heat.
7. Grill the veggies for 15 to 20 minutes while flipping them every 5 minutes.
8. Blend all the vinaigrette ingredients together in a small bowl.
9. Put the grilled veggies and the cooked quinoa in a bowl or container.
10. Top it with a scoop of cooked black beans and some vinaigrette.
11. Enjoy or store for another day!

STORAGE INFORMATION:

Storage	Temperature	Expiration date	Preparation
3-compartment airtight container M/L	Fridge at 38 – 40°F or 3°C	2-3 days after preparation	Reheat in microwave
3-compartment airtight container M/L	Freezer at -1°F or -20°C	60 days after preparation	Thaw at room temperature. Reheat in microwave

Note: Keep the black beans separated from the vinaigrette and the quinoa mixed with the veggies. Use one container with multiple compartments or separate containers for storage.

15. Spicy Mediterranean Hummus

Serves: 12 | Prep Time: ~25 min |

Total number of Ingredients: 11

Nutrition Information
(per serving)

- Calories: 137 kcal.
- Carbs: 13g.
- Fat: 7.8g.
- Protein: 5g.
- Fiber: 3.4g.
- Sugar: 2g.

INGREDIENTS:

- 3 cups dry chickpeas
- 3 tbsp. olive oil
- 5 tbsp. tahini
- 1 cup water
- 5 cloves garlic (minced)
- 3 tbsp. lemon juice
- 1 tsp. cumin
- ½ tsp. cayenne pepper
- Salt and pepper to taste
- ¼ cup fresh cilantro or parsley
  (optional, chopped)
- ¼ cup red pepper bell (optional,
  medium, diced)

METHOD

1. Prepare the chickpeas according to the recipe.
2. Add the cooked chickpeas, tahini, olive oil and the water to a blender.
3. Blend until the mixture is smooth.
4. Add the garlic, lemon juice, cumin, cayenne pepper and a pinch of salt.
5. Blend the hummus again until all ingredients are incorporated and the hummus is smooth.
6. Transfer the hummus to a container. Top it with some additional pepper and salt to taste.
7. Serve with fresh chopped cilantro, parsley or diced red pepper bell on top.
8. Enjoy, share or store!

STORAGE INFORMATION:

Storage	Temperature	Expiration date	Preparation
Airtight container M	Fridge at 38 – 40°F or 3°C	4-5 days after preparation	
Airtight container M	Freezer at -1°F or -20°C	60 days after preparation	Thaw at room temperature.

16. Cheezy Quinoa

Total number of Ingredients: 9

Nutrition Information
(per serving)
- Calories: 259 kcal.
- Carbs: 30.8g.
- Fat: 11.4g.
- Protein: 8.6g.
- Fiber: 3.6g.
- Sugar: 2g.

INGREDIENTS:

- 3 cups dry quinoa
- 1 butternut squash (small, seeded, cubed)
- ¼ cup almond milk (unsweetened)
- 1 tbsp. Dijon mustard
- 3 tbsp. flour
- 5 grates fresh nutmeg
- 1 cup cashew cheese spread (page 52)
- ¼ cup arugula (chopped)
- Salt and pepper to taste

METHOD

1. Preheat the oven to 350°F or 175°C.
2. Prepare the quinoa according to the recipe.
3. Take a medium pot, fill it with water and bring it to boil.
4. Boil the cubed butternut squash in this water on medium heat for about 15 minutes.
5. Drain the squash and transfer it to a blender.
6. Blend the squash while adding the almond milk and Dijon mustard until it's a thick creamy sauce.
7. Add the flour and nutmeg.
8. Pour the blended ingredients into a large bowl.
9. Add the cooked quinoa and vegan cheese to the mix and stir well.
10. Transfer the mixture to a baking dish lined with parchment paper and bake the mixture for about 20 minutes in the oven until it has a bubbly texture.
11. Serve the cheezy quinoa on a plate with arugula on top and add more salt and pepper to taste.
12. Serve or store for later!

STORAGE INFORMATION:

Storage	Temperature	Expiration date	Preparation
Airtight container M/L	Fridge at 38 – 40°F or 3°C	2-3 days after preparation	Reheat in microwave
Airtight container M/L	Freezer at -1°F or -20°C	60 days after preparation	Thaw at room temperature. Reheat in microwave

17. Roasted Green Beans & Basil

Serves: 2 | Prep Time: ~20 min |

Total number of Ingredients: 9

Nutrition Information
(per serving)
- Calories: 338 kcal.
- Carbs: 6.9g.
- Fat: 32.4g.
- Protein 4.9g.
- Fiber: 3.4g.
- Sugar: 1.1g.

INGREDIENTS:
- 3 tbsp. olive oil
- 2 cups green beans (whole)
- ½ tbsp. basil (dried)
- ½ cup raw almonds (crushed)
- 1 tsp. lemon zest
- 1 tbsp. lemon juice
- 2 garlic cloves (minced)
- Salt and pepper to taste
- Fresh basil (optional)

METHOD
1. Preheat the oven to 450°F or 225°C.
2. Grease a large baking tray with the olive oil.
3. Put all the ingredients except the optional fresh basil on the tray and stir until all the ingredients are greased.
4. Roast the food in the oven for about 20 minutes.
5. Garnish the roasted mix with the optional fresh basil.
6. Serve and enjoy or store for another day!

STORAGE INFORMATION:

Storage	Temperature	Expiration date	Preparation
Airtight container M/L	Fridge at 38 – 40°F or 3°C	4-5 days after preparation	Reheat in pot or microwave
Airtight container M/L	Freezer at -1°F or -20°C	60 days after preparation	Thaw at room temperature. Reheat in pot or microwave

Tip: Keep the optional fresh basil in the original package and take out a portion on the day of consumption.

18. Roasted Bell Pepper Hummus

Serves: 12 | Prep Time: ~25 min |

Total number of Ingredients: 8

Nutrition Information
(per serving)
- Calories: 97 kcal.
- Carbs: 13g.
- Fat: 3g.
- Protein: 4.6g.
- Fiber: 3.5g.
- Sugar: 2.5g.

INGREDIENTS:
- 3 cups of dry chickpeas
- 3 tbsp. olive oil
- 3 tbsp. tahini
- ½ cup water
- 1 red bell pepper (seeded, diced)
- 3 tbsp. lemon juice (more to taste)
- ½ tsp. cumin
- Salt and pepper to taste

METHOD
1. Preheat oven to 400°F or 200°C.
2. Prepare the chickpeas according to the recipe.
3. Add most of the cooked chickpeas, olive oil, tahini and the water to a blender.
4. Blend the ingredients for 1-2 minutes until smooth.
5. Broil the red bell pepper slices in the oven on a tray for about 10 minutes.
6. Allow the roasted red bell pepper slices to cool.
7. Throw the red bell pepper slices and the other remaining ingredients into the blender.
8. Blend all the ingredients until all ingredients are incorporated and the hummus is smooth.
9. Transfer the hummus to a container and top it with some additional olive oil, cooked chickpeas and salt and pepper to taste.
10. Enjoy, share or store for later!

STORAGE INFORMATION:

Storage	Temperature	Expiration date	Preparation
Airtight container M/L	Fridge at 38 – 40°F or 3°C	4-5 days after preparation	
Airtight container M/L	Freezer at -1°F or -20°C	60 days after preparation	Thaw at room temperature.

DINNER RECIPES

1. Triple Bean Chili

Total number of Ingredients: 18

Nutrition Information
(per serving)
- Calories: 143 kcal.
- Carbs: 23g.
- Fat: 3.5g.
- Protein: 5.9g.
- Fiber: 9.6g.
- Sugar: 4.4g.

INGREDIENTS:
- ½ cup raw black beans
- ½ cup raw kidney beans
- ½ cup raw chickpeas
- 4 tomatoes (medium, sliced)
- 1½ tbsp. olive oil
- 1 onion (large, diced)
- 1 cup mushrooms (chopped)
- 4 cloves garlic (minced)
- 2 tbsp. chili powder
- 2 tsp. cumin
- 1 tsp. dried oregano
- 1 tsp. thyme
- Salt and black pepper to taste
- 1 red bell pepper (medium, diced)
- 2 cups vegetable broth (page 63)
- 1 bay leaf
- 1 (200g.) can sweet corn
- 1 lime (juiced)

METHOD
1. Preheat the oven to 400°F or 200°C.
2. Prepare the black and kidney beans according to the recipe.
3. Prepare the chickpeas according to the recipe.
4. Lay out the sliced tomatoes on a baking sheet lined with parchment paper. Drizzle the slices with half of the olive oil and a pinch of salt.
5. Put the tray with tomatoes in the oven for about 10 minutes.
6. Take a large pan, put it on medium heat and add the remaining olive oil.
7. Sauté the onions with some black pepper for about 5 minutes.
8. Add in the mushrooms and minced garlic.
9. Stir well and heat the mixture for another 5 minutes.
10. Add the chili powder, cumin, oregano, thyme, salt and more pepper to the mix.
11. Stir for 1 minute and add the vegetable broth, red bell pepper, roasted tomatoes, cooked beans and chickpeas, corn and bay leaf.
12. Turn the heat to medium and allow the chili to cook for about a minute.
13. Now turn the heat to low, cover the pot and let the mixture simmer for about 20 minutes.
14. Remove the pot from the heat.
15. Serve the meal in a bowl with some fresh lime juice on top.
16. Enjoy warm or allow the chili to cool before storage!

STORAGE INFORMATION:

Storage	Temperature	Expiration date	Preparation
Airtight container M/L	Fridge at 38 – 40°F or 3°C	3-4 days after preparation	Reheat in microwave
Airtight container M/L	Freezer at -1°F or -20°C	60 days after preparation	Thaw at room temperature. Reheat in microwave

2. Vegan Goulash

Serves: 5 | Prep Time: ~45 min |

Total number of Ingredients: 12

Nutrition Information
(per serving)

- Calories: 591 kcal.
- Carbs: 83.8g.
- Fat: 18.7g.
- Protein: 16.5g.
- Fiber: 14.2g.
- Sugar: 20.4g.

INGREDIENTS:

- 5 tbsp. olive oil
- 12 onions (medium, finely chopped)
- 1 head garlic (minced)
- 4 red bell peppers (cored, chopped)
- 10 tomatoes (small, cubed)
- 4 tbsp. paprika powder
- ½ cup dry red wine
- 3-6 cups vegetable broth (page 63)
- 10 potatoes (medium, skinned, cubed)
- 1 (7oz.) pack tempeh (substitute with textured soy protein)
- Salt and pepper to taste
- ¼ cup fresh parsley (chopped)

METHOD

1. Heat the olive oil, in a large pot over medium heat.
2. Sauté the onions until brown.
3. Add the minced garlic and stir for 1 minute.
4. Continue to add the chopped bell peppers and cook the ingredients for another 3 minutes while stirring.
5. Blend in the tomatoes, paprika powder, salt, pepper and the dry red wine.
6. Stir thoroughly while letting the mixture cook for another 2 minutes.
7. Add the vegetable broth and the potato cubes to the pot and stir to combine all ingredients.
8. Put a lid on the pot and allow the goulash to cook for another 5 minutes.
9. Turn the heat down to low and continue to gently cook the goulash for 15 minutes. The goulash will thicken and the potatoes will get cooked properly.
10. Add the tempeh and taste to see if the goulash needs more salt and pepper.
11. Let the goulash cook for another 15 minutes.
12. Check if the potatoes have softened with a fork. Cook the mixture a few minutes more if the potatoes are hard to penetrate.
13. Once the potatoes are soft, add the parsley, stir and take the goulash off the heat.
14. Allow the goulash to cool down for about 10 minutes and serve or allow the goulash to cool down longer before storing.

STORAGE INFORMATION:

Storage	Temperature	Expiration date	Preparation
Airtight container M/L	Fridge at 38 – 40°F or 3°C	3-4 days after preparation	Reheat in microwave
Airtight container M/L	Freezer at -1°F or -20°C	60 days after preparation	Thaw at room temperature. Reheat in microwave

3. Tempeh Curry

Serves: 4 | Prep Time: ~ 20 min |

Total number of Ingredients: 17

Nutrition Information
(per serving)
- Calories: 411 kcal.
- Carbs: 44.5g.
- Fat: 13.7g.
- Protein: 27.5g.
- Fiber: 8.4g.
- Sugar: 4.4g.

INGREDIENTS:
- 15 oz. tempeh
- 2 cups quinoa
- ½ cup red bell pepper (chopped)
- ½ cup purple cabbage (shredded)
- ½ cup sweet potato (finely chopped)
- 2 cups kale (chopped)
- 2 cups broccoli florets (chopped, fresh or frozen)

Tempeh seasoning:
- 3 tbsp. soy sauce
- 3 tbsp. sesame oil
- 3 tsp. rice vinegar
- 1 tsp. chili flakes (optional)

Cashew Curry Sauce:
- ½ cup cashew cheese spread (page 52)
- ¼ cup coconut cream
- ¼ cup coconut milk
- 2 tbsp. soy sauce
- 3 tsp. rice vinegar
- 2 tsp. red curry paste

METHOD
1. Prepare the quinoa according to the recipe.
2. Use a sharp cutting knife to cut the tempeh into small, thin squares.
3. Transfer the tempeh squares to a medium sized bowl.
4. Marinate the squares with soy sauce, sesame oil and rice vinegar.
5. Carefully stir the tempeh and allow the squares to sit in the seasoning for 10 minutes.
6. Stir-fry the marinated tempeh in a large skillet with the chopped bell pepper, cabbage and sweet potato for about 5 minutes.
7. Take the skillet off the heat and set the stir-fried tempeh and veggies aside.
8. Fill a large pot with water and bring it to a boil.
9. Steam or cook the chopped broccoli florets in a sieve for about 3 minutes and set aside.
10. Reuse the large pot and add all the curry sauce ingredients.
11. Put the pot on low heat and gently whisk the ingredients until a smooth creamy sauce has formed.
12. Stir in the freshly chopped kale, cooked broccoli, fried tempeh and veggies.
13. Add the quinoa to the curry mixture in the pot and mix.
14. Enjoy warm or store for later!

STORAGE INFORMATION:

Storage	Temperature	Expiration date	Preparation
Airtight container M/L	Fridge at 38 – 40°F or 3°C	2-3 days after preparation	Reheat in microwave
Airtight container M/L	Freezer at -1°F or -20°C	60 days after preparation	Thaw at room temperature. Reheat in microwave

4. Quinoa and Broccoli Stew

Serves: 4 | Prep Time: ~ 30 min |

Total number of Ingredients: 12

Nutrition Information
(per serving)
- Calories: 326 kcal.
- Carbs: 47g.
- Fat: 10g.
- Protein: 12g.
- Fiber: 20.5g.
- Sugar: 11g.

INGREDIENTS:

- 2 cups cooked quinoa
- 2 tbsp. olive oil
- 3 cloves garlic (minced)
- 1 yellow bell pepper (seeded, diced)
- 1 red bell pepper (seeded, diced)
- 3 carrots (diced)
- 2 sweet potatoes (skinned, diced)
- 3 cups broccoli florets (roughly chopped)
- 2 cups almond milk (unsweetened)
- 2 bay leaves
- 2 tsp. thyme
- Salt and pepper to taste

METHOD

1. Prepare the quinoa according to the recipe.
2. Put a large pot on medium heat.
3. Add the olive oil to the pot and stir-fry the minced garlic for about 1 minute until caramelized.
4. Add the red and yellow bell peppers and fry all ingredients for 8-10 minutes.
5. Continue to add the carrots, sweet potatoes, broccoli florets, almond milk, bay leaves, thyme and salt.
6. Bring the mixture to a boil. Turn the heat down after a minute to low and allow the ingredients to gently cook for another 10-12 minutes to soften the broccoli and sweet potatoes.
7. Lower the heat and allow the broccoli stew to cool a bit.
8. Put half of the stew without the bay leaves in a blender and blend until soft.
9. Transfer the blended stew back to the pot with the original half and stir again.
10. Make sure the prepared quinoa is drained well.
11. Remove the bay leaves from the stew, stir the cooked quinoa in and cook the mix for another 3 minutes on medium heat. The quinoa will absorb excess liquid and thicken the stew.
12. Turn off heat and allow the stew to cool before serving or storing.

STORAGE INFORMATION:

Storage	Temperature	Expiration date	Preparation
Airtight container M/L	Fridge at 38 – 40°F or 3°C	2-3 days after preparation	Reheat in microwave
Airtight container M/L	Freezer at -1°F or -20°C	60 days after preparation	Thaw at room temperature. Reheat in microwave

5. Crunchy Sesame Tofu

Serves: 2 | Prep Time: ~15 min |

Total number of Ingredients: 13

Nutrition Information
(per serving)
- Calories: 654 kcal.
- Carbs 35.4g.
- Fat: 41.9.
- Protein: 33.9g.
- Fiber: 9.1g.
- Sugar: 22g.

INGREDIENTS:
- 3 tbsp. sesame oil
- 2 cups firm tofu (cubed)
- ¼ cup soy sauce
- 2 zucchinis (medium, sliced into noodles)
- 2 tbsp. roasted sesame seeds (optional)
- 1 green onion (sliced, optional)

Sesame peanut topping:
- ½ cup peanut butter
- ¼ cup soy sauce
- ¼ cup rice vinegar
- 2 tsp. chili flakes
- 2 tbsp. maple syrup
- 5g. of fresh ginger (peeled, chopped)
- 3 garlic cloves

METHOD
1. Put a large skillet on medium heat and add 2 tablespoons of sesame oil.
2. Put in the cubed tofu and sauté these until light brown.
3. Add the first ¼ cup of soy sauce and stir well.
4. Turn the heat down to low and allow the tofu to absorb the soy sauce until the tofu is slightly crisp.
5. Put the crispy tofu aside for later.
6. Take a blender and mix all the sesame peanut topping ingredients.
7. Mix the tofu with the sesame peanut topping.
8. Serve the raw zucchini noodles with the crispy tofu and sauce in a medium bowl.
9. Top the dish with the optional roasted sesame seeds and green onion slices.
10. Serve and enjoy right away or store the ingredients separately!

STORAGE INFORMATION:

Storage	Temperature	Expiration date	Preparation
3-section airtight container M/L or/ and Ziploc bags	Fridge at 38 – 40°F or 3°C	4-5 days after preparation	Reheat in pot or microwave
3-section airtight container M/L or/ and Ziploc bags	Freezer at -1°F or -20°C	60 days after preparation	Thaw at room temperature. Reheat in pot or microwave

Note: Keep the zucchini noodles, tofu and toppings in a 3 or 4-section container, separate containers and/ or Ziploc bags.

6. Golden Tofu Noodle Bowl

Serves: 2 | Prep Time: ~15 min |

Total number of Ingredients: 13

Nutrition Information
(per serving)
- Calories: 547 kcal.
- Carbs: 63.3g.
- Fat: 22.4.
- Protein: 23.3g.
- Fiber: 9.3g.
- Sugar: 12.7g.

INGREDIENTS:

- 1½ cups brown rice or rice noodles
- 1 cup firm tofu (cubed)
- 2 tbsp. coconut oil
- 1 radish (sliced)
- 1 carrot (large, peeled)
- ½ cucumber (sliced)
- 1 cup edamame (shelled)
- ¼ cup pickled red cabbage (optional)
- Roasted sesame seeds (optional)

Soy hoisin sauce:
- 3 tbsp. hoisin sauce
- 1 tsp. sriracha (or tabasco)
- ¼ cup soy sauce
- 1 lime (squeezed)

METHOD

1. Cook the rice (or noodles) according to the recipe or package instructions.
2. Put in all sauce ingredients into a small bowl and stir well. Set the sauce aside.
3. Boil some water in a medium pot.
4. Steam the edamame in a sieve above the boiling water for about 5 minutes and shell them.
5. Take a large skillet, put it on medium heat and add the coconut oil.
6. Stir fry the tofu for about 5 minutes until brown before stirring in the hoisin sauce.
7. Serve the cooked rice or noodles with the tofu and sauce in a bowl.
8. Top the dish with the steamed edamame, carrot, cucumber and raw radish.
9. Add the optional roasted sesame seeds and pickled red cabbage.
10. Serve and enjoy or store the fresh and cooked ingredients in multiple-compartment containers!

STORAGE INFORMATION:

Storage	Temperature	Expiration date	Preparation
3-section airtight container M/L or/ and Ziploc bags	Fridge at 38 – 40°F or 3°C	4-5 days after preparation	Reheat in pot or microwave
3-section airtight container M/L or/ and Ziploc bags	Freezer at -1°F or -20°C	60 days after preparation	Thaw at room temperature. Reheat in pot or microwave

Note: Store the rice, tofu and vegetables in 3-section containers or separate containers. Serve the meal with some extra (fresh or pre-made) soy hoisin sauce to add more flavor!

7. Broccoli Quiche

Serves: 4 | Prep Time: ~25 min |

Total number of Ingredients: 11

Nutrition Information
(per serving)
- Calories: 378 kcal.
- Carbs: 43.1g.
- Fat: 19g.
- Protein: 8.8g.
- Fiber: 13.4g.
- Sugar: 5.5g.

INGREDIENTS:

- 1 pre-made vegan pie crust (page 59)
- 1 tbsp. olive oil
- 2 cups broccoli florets (chopped)
- 1 onion (large, diced)
- 1 green bell pepper (chopped)
- 1 cup fresh mushrooms (quartered)
- 1 tsp. nutmeg
- ½ tsp. turmeric
- 1 tbsp. basil
- ½ cup almond milk
- Salt and pepper to taste

METHOD

1. Prepare the pie crust uncooked according to the recipe (page 59) in a cake tin.
2. Heat the oven to 350°F or 175°C.
3. Take a large saucepan and put it on medium heat.
4. Add the olive oil and diced onions. Sauté the onions for a few minutes until browned.
5. Continue to add the mushrooms, bell pepper and broccoli florets.
6. Lower the heat and keep stirring for about 5 minutes.
7. Whisk the nutmeg, turmeric, basil, salt and almond milk in a cup until smooth.
8. Combine the almond milk mixture with the veggies in the saucepan.
9. Take the saucepan off the heat and pour the veggie mixture into the prepared pie crust.
10. Cover the quiche with aluminum foil and bake it in the oven for about 30 minutes until browned.
11. Allow the quiche to cool down before serving or storing.

STORAGE INFORMATION:

Storage	Temperature	Expiration date	Preparation
Airtight container M/L or Ziploc bag	Fridge at 38 – 40°F or 3°C	2-3 days after preparation	Reheat in pot or microwave
Airtight container M/L or Ziploc bag	Freezer at -1°F or -20°C	60 days after preparation	Thaw at room temperature. Reheat in pot or microwave

8. Vegan Falafel Balls

Total number of Ingredients: 10

Nutrition Information
(per serving)
- Calories: 64 kcal.
- Carbs: 7g.
- Fat: 2.7g.
- Protein: 2.9g.
- Fiber: 3.7g.
- Sugar: 0.9g.

INGREDIENTS:

- 2 cups dry chickpeas
- ½ cup parsley (chopped, fresh)
- ¾ cup white onions (minced)
- 4 cloves garlic (medium, minced)
- 2 tbsp. sesame seeds (raw)
- 1½ tsp. cumin
- ¼ tsp. salt and pepper (or to taste)
- 3 tbsp. whole wheat flour (more or less, depending on the batter's consistency)
- Brown bread crumbs for coating (optional)
- ¼ cup olive oil

METHOD

1. Cook chickpeas according to the recipe.
2. Add the cooked chickpeas, parsley, onion, garlic, sesame seeds, cumin, salt and pepper to a blender or food processor. Blend the ingredients into a crumbly-looking dough. Prevent blending too long, resulting in a smooth paste.
3. Take out the dough and transfer it to a flat surface covered with a tea towel.
4. Add about a tablespoon of flour at a time and knead the dough into a non-sticky mix.
5. Place the mixture into a medium bowl. Cover the bowl and refrigerate it for 2 hours or until the dough is firm.
6. Scoop out rounded tablespoon amounts and form into small balls. When using the optional bread crumbs, sprinkle them on and lightly press them to both sides of the scooped amounts.
7. Put a large skillet on medium heat, add olive oil and wait until the oil is hot. Add as many falafels as possible to the pan and bake them for about 5 minutes. Make sure to cook both sides.
8. The falafels will be complete when both sides are golden brown and crisp.
9. Allow the falafels to cool. Serve with vegan garlic sauce or mayo (page 60). Alternatively store the falafels for later.

STORAGE INFORMATION:

Storage	Temperature	Expiration date	Preparation
Airtight container M	Fridge at 38 – 40°F or 3°C	3-4 days after preparation	Reheat in pot or microwave
Airtight container M	Freezer at -1°F or -20°C	60 days after preparation	Thaw at room temperature. Reheat in pot or microwave

9. Spicy Beet Bowl

Total number of Ingredients: 16

Nutrition Information
(per serving)

- Calories: 445 kcal.
- Carbs: 48.7g.
- Fat: 20.5g.
- Protein: 16.4g.
- Fiber: 17.3g.
- Sugar: 14.2g.

INGREDIENTS:

Bowl contents:

- 1 cup dry sushi rice
- 3 Chioggia beets (medium, sliced)
- ¼ lemon (fresh, juice)
- 2-4 tsp. olive oil
- 2g. fresh ginger (peeled, cut)
- 2 cups edamame beans
- 2 tsp. olive oil
- 2 green onions (sliced)
- 1 carrot (big, sliced)
- Salt to taste
- 3 tsp. roasted sesame seeds (optional)
- Handful nori flakes (optional)

Wasabi avocado paste:

- 1 avocado (big, peeled and pitted)
- ¼ lemon (fresh, juice)
- 2 tsp. wasabi powder
- Salt to taste

METHOD

1. Preheat oven to 375°F or 190°C.
2. Cook the sushi rice according to the recipe.
3. Wrap the sliced Chioggia beets in aluminum foil.
4. Transfer the packed beet slices to a baking tray and put it in the oven.
5. Roast the beets for about 45 minutes. Take the tray out and set it aside.
6. Scoop out the avocado flesh and cut it into small pieces.
7. Transfer the avocado to a small bowl and add half of the lemon juice, wasabi powder and salt to taste.
8. Mash until the avocado mixture is creamy and set aside.
9. Take a large bowl and mix in the other half of the lemon juice, olive oil, ginger and more salt to taste.
10. Take the foil off the roasted beets and put the slices in this large bowl.
11. Boil some water in a medium pot.
12. Steam the edamame beans topped with a pinch of salt in a sieve above the boiling water for about 5 minutes.
13. Top the edamame with a pinch of olive oil and salt to taste. Set the beans aside.
14. Take a medium bowl for serving and add the rice, beets and steamed edamame.
15. Top the dish with the wasabi avocado paste, green onion slices, carrot slices, optional roasted sesame seeds and nori flakes.
16. Serve and enjoy or store the ingredients separately for another day!

STORAGE INFORMATION:

Storage	Temperature	Expiration date	Preparation
4-section airtight container and/ or Ziploc bags	Fridge at 38 – 40°F or 3°C	2 days after preparation	Reheat in pot or microwave and add toppings after heating.
4-section airtight container and/ or Ziploc bags	Freezer at -1°F or -20°C	60 days after preparation	Thaw at room temperature. Reheat in pot or microwave and add toppings after heating.

Note: Keep the rice, roasted beet slices, vegetables and the avocado wasabi paste in a 4-section container, separate containers and/or Ziploc bags.

10. Veggie Poke Bowl

Serves: 2 | Prep Time: ~15 min |

Total number of Ingredients: 14

Nutrition Information
(per serving)
- Calories: 401 kcal.
- Carbs: 45.5g.
- Fat: 18.6g.
- Protein 13.1.
- Fiber: 6.2g.
- Sugar: 15g.

INGREDIENTS:

Vegan stir fry sauce:
- 3 tbsp. soy sauce
- 3 tbsp. water
- 2 tbsp. brown sugar
- 1 tsp. sriracha (or tabasco sauce)
- ½ tsp. sesame oil

Avocado wasabi paste:
- 1 avocado (mashed)
- 1 tsp. wasabi paste

Bowl contents:
- 1 cup dry white rice
- 1 tsp. sesame oil
- 1 cup extra firm tofu (cubed or sliced)
- 1 tsp. red pepper flakes
- 1 tsp. pickled ginger
- 1 green onion (medium, chopped)
- Roasted sesame seeds (optional)

METHOD

1. Cook the white rice according to the recipe.
2. Mix all the vegan stir-fry sauce ingredients in a small bowl and stir well.
3. Grease a large skillet with 1 teaspoon of sesame oil and put it on medium heat.
4. Add the stir-fry sauce and tofu. Stir-fry the tofu for about 5 minutes.
5. Continue to add the red pepper flakes and turn the heat down to low.
6. Take another small bowl and mix the avocado and wasabi paste.
7. Serve the cooked rice and stir-fried tofu in a medium bowl.
8. Top the dish with the avocado and wasabi paste, pickled ginger, green onion and the optional roasted sesame seeds.
9. Serve or store the prepared ingredients separately!

STORAGE INFORMATION:

Storage	Temperature	Expiration date	Preparation
3-section airtight container M/L and/or Ziploc bags	Fridge at 38 – 40°F or 3°C	2-3 days after preparation	Reheat in pot or microwave
3-section airtight container M/L and/or Ziploc bags	Freezer at -1°F or -20°C	60 days after preparation	Thaw at room temperature. Reheat in pot or microwave

Note: Store the rice, tofu and vegetables in a 3-section container. Alternatively, use separate containers and/or Ziploc bags. Serve this dish with extra spices to taste.

11. Bean Burritos

Total number of Ingredients: 18

Nutrition Information
(per serving)
- Calories: 408 kcal.
- Carbs: 76.25g.
- Fat: 11.4g.
- Protein: 14.5g.
- Fiber: 14.4g.
- Sugar: 4.6g.

INGREDIENTS:
- ½ cup dry black beans
- 1 cup dry quinoa
- 4 tortillas (large, whole wheat)
- 2 tbsp. olive oil
- 3 cloves garlic (minced)
- 1 zucchini (medium, quartered vertically)
- 1 green bell pepper (medium, pitted, diced)
- 1 tomato (medium, diced)
- 1 (100g) can sweet corn (drained)
- 1 tbsp. fresh lime juice
- Salt and pepper to taste

Optional: special spiced pesto
- 1 cup cilantro leaves
- ¼ cup cashews (raw)
- ¼ cup olive oil
- 1 clove garlic
- 1 jalapeño pepper (small, seeded)
- 1 tbsp. lime juice
- Salt and pepper to taste

METHOD
1. Prepare the black beans according to the recipe.
2. Cook the quinoa according to the recipe.
3. Put a large skillet on medium heat and add the olive oil.
4. Add the garlic, zucchini and bell pepper.
5. Stir the vegetables for about 10 minutes while adding the tomato and corn.
6. Transfer the vegetables to a large bowl.
7. Top the veggies with salt and black pepper to taste and stir well.
8. Prepare the optional pesto by blending all the special spiced pesto ingredients in a blender or food processor.
9. Top the veggies in the bowl with the optional pesto and stir well for about 2 minutes.
10. Scoop a portion of cooked beans and quinoa onto a tortilla.
11. Add some of the vegetable mixture with the optional pesto to the tortilla.
12. Top the mixture with some fresh lime juice.
13. Wrap the tortilla tightly and enjoy or store!

STORAGE INFORMATION:

Storage	Temperature	Expiration date	Preparation
Airtight container M/L or aluminum foil.	Fridge at 38 – 40°F or 3°C	3-4 days after preparation	Reheat in microwave
Airtight container M/L or aluminum foil.	Freezer at -1°F or -20°C	60 days after preparation	Thaw at room temperature. Reheat in microwave

Note: Wrap each prepared burrito in aluminum foil before storing in a storage container or Ziploc bag. WARNING: Do NOT microwave aluminum foil!

12. 'Veggieful' Chili

Serves: 8 | Prep Time: ~15 min |

Total number of Ingredients: 17

Nutrition Information
(per serving)

- Calories: 256 kcal.
- Carbs: 43.6g.
- Fat: 4.5gr.
- Protein: 13g.
- Fiber: 16.8g.
- Sugar: 8.5g.

INGREDIENTS:

- 1½ cups raw black beans
- 1½ cups raw kidney beans
- 2 tbsp. olive oil
- 2 red onions (medium, diced)
- 1 clove garlic (minced)
- 2 tsp. cumin
- ¼ tsp. cayenne pepper
- 2 tsp. oregano
- 1 zucchini (medium, diced)
- 1 yellow squash (small, diced)
- 1 red bell pepper (small, diced)
- 2 cups water
- 1 jalapeño (medium, diced)
- 1 cup tomato paste
- 1 (200g) can sweet corn (drained)
- 1 tbsp. chili powder
- Salt and pepper to taste

METHOD

1. Prepare the black and kidney beans according to the recipe.
2. Take a large pan, put it on medium high heat and add the olive oil.
3. Sautee the diced red onions for about 5 minutes.
4. Blend in the garlic, cumin, cayenne pepper, oregano while stirring.
5. Add the diced zucchini, squash, bell pepper and stir again.
6. Allow the mixture to fry for a few minutes while constantly stirring.
7. Lower the heat to medium and add 2 cups of water, jalapeño, tomato paste, corn and cooked beans.
8. Stir well while adding the chili powder, salt and optionally more pepper to taste.
9. Reduce the heat to low, cover the pan and let the chili simmer for about 20 minutes.
10. Add more spices like cumin, oregano, chili powder or cayenne pepper to taste.
11. Serve and enjoy warm or allow the chili to cool down to store it in containers!

STORAGE INFORMATION:

Storage	Temperature	Expiration date	Preparation
2-compartment airtight container M	Fridge at 38 – 40°F or 3°C	3-4 days after preparation	Reheat in microwave
2-compartment airtight container M	Freezer at -1°F or -20°C	60 days after preparation	Thaw at room temperature. Reheat in microwave

Note: Keep the black beans separated from the chili. Use a 2-compartment or two separate containers to store each meal.

13. Red Curry Lentils

Serves: 6 | Prep Time: ~20 min|

Total number of Ingredients: 14

Nutrition Information
(per serving)
- Calories: 162 kcal.
- Carbs: 19.3g.
- Fat: 6.8g.
- Protein: 6g.
- Fiber: 6.5g.
- Sugar: 5.8g.

INGREDIENTS:
- 1 cup dry red lentils
- 2 tbsp. coconut oil
- 1 tbsp. cumin seeds
- 1 tbsp. coriander seeds
- 8 tomatoes (ripe, cubed)
- 1 head of garlic (chopped or minced)
- 2 tbsp. ginger (chopped)
- 1 tbsp. turmeric
- 1 tsp. cayenne powder
- 3 cups vegetable broth (page 63)
- 2 tsp. sea salt
- 1 (15oz.) can coconut milk
- ½ cup cherry tomatoes
- ½ cup cilantro (chopped)

METHOD
1. Soak and drain the red lentils according to the recipe but do not cook them yet.
2. Put the coconut oil in a large pot heating over medium high heat.
3. Add the cumin and coriander seeds and garlic. Sauté the ingredients for about 2 minutes while continuously stirring.
4. Add the freshly cut tomato cubes, ginger, turmeric and a pinch of salt to the pot.
5. Allow the mixture to gently cook, stirring occasionally for 5 minutes.
6. Blend in the red lentils, more salt to taste and cayenne powder.
7. Continue to add 3 cups of vegetable broth to the pot and allow the mixture to come to a soft boil.
8. Reduce the heat to low, cover the pot and allow the dish to simmer for about 30 minutes while stirring occasionally.
9. Once the lentils are soft, add the coconut milk and cherry tomatoes.
10. Bring the mixture back to a simmer before removing it from the heat and stir in the chopped cilantro.
11. Serve warm or allow the curry to cool down before storing.

STORAGE INFORMATION:

Storage	Temperature	Expiration date	Preparation
Airtight container M/L	Fridge at 38 – 40°F or 3°C	3-4 days after preparation	Reheat in pot or microwave
Airtight container M/L	Freezer at -1°F or -20°C	60 days after preparation	Thaw at room temperature. Reheat in pot or microwave

Note: Enjoy the curry with some rice on the side!

14. Black-Bean Veggie Burritos

Total number of Ingredients: 21

Nutrition Information
(per serving)
- Calories: 285 kcal.
- Carbs: 40.9g.
- Fat: 9.8g.
- Protein: 8.6g.
- Fiber: 6.7g.
- Sugar: 4.3g.

INGREDIENTS:

For the filling:
- 2 cups dry black beans
- 1 tbsp. olive oil
- 1 red onion (diced)
- 1 zucchini (cubed)
- 1 red bell pepper (pitted, diced)
- 2 (150g) cans sweet corn (drained, rinsed)
- ¼ cup cilantro (chopped)
- ½ a lime (juiced)
- Salt to taste

For homemade taco seasoning (optional)
- 1 tbsp. chili powder
- 2 tsp. ground cumin
- ½ tsp. paprika powder
- ¼ tsp. of each: garlic powder, onion powder, red pepper flakes, oregano, salt and cayenne

For the wraps:
- 8 tortilla wraps (page 67)
- ½ cup no-salt vegan cream cheese (page 61)
- ½ cup salsa (page 49)
- 1 cup dry brown rice

METHOD

1. Cook the black beans according to the recipe.
2. Prepare the brown rice according to the recipe.
3. Mix all taco seasoning ingredients in a bowl and set it aside.
4. Take a large pan, add the olive oil and put it on medium heat.
5. Add the diced red onion. Sauté for 3 minutes while stirring.
6. Add the zucchini and bell pepper and sauté for another 3 minutes.
7. Add in the black beans, corn and the homemade taco seasoning. Stir well and allow the mixture to simmer for about 10 minutes.
8. Turn off the heat and add the cilantro, lime juice and salt to taste.
9. Prepare the burrito by laying out a tortilla wrap and add the filling, salsa, rice and the optional vegan cheese.
10. Tightly wrap the burrito and place it back in the pan. Heat and press each side for about 2 minutes.
11. Serve warm or store each tortilla wrapped in aluminum foil in a Ziploc bag.

STORAGE INFORMATION:

Storage	Temperature	Expiration date	Preparation
Ziploc bag, wrapped in aluminum foil	Fridge at 38 – 40°F or 3°C	3-4 days after preparation	Reheat in pot or microwave
Ziploc bag, wrapped in aluminum foil	Freezer at -1°F or -20°C	60 days after preparation	Thaw at room temperature. Reheat in pot or microwave

15. Baked Red Bell Peppers

Serves: 8 | Prep Time: ~30 min |

Total number of Ingredients: 14

Nutrition Information
(per serving)

- Calories: 135 kcal.
- Carbs: 20g.
- Fat: 4g.
- Protein: 4.5g.
- Fiber: 16.4g.
- Sugar: 5.5g.

INGREDIENTS:

- 1 cup dry chickpeas
- 1½ cup dry quinoa
- 4 red bell peppers (seeded, halved lengthwise)
- 1½ tbsp. olive oil
- 1 red onion (medium, diced)
- 1 clove garlic (medium, minced)
- 2 tbsp. chili powder
- 2 tsp. cumin
- 1 tsp. cayenne pepper
- 2 tsp. spicy paprika powder
- 2 cups baby spinach (chopped)
- 3 tomatoes (ripe, medium, chopped)
- ¼ cup fresh cilantro (chopped)
- Salt and pepper to taste

METHOD

1. Preheat the oven to 375°F or 190°C.
2. Prepare the chickpeas according to the recipe.
3. Prepare the quinoa according to the recipe.
4. Put the olive oil into a skillet on medium heat.
5. Sautee the diced red onions until soft.
6. Add the garlic, chili powder, cumin, cayenne pepper, paprika powder, salt and pepper to the skillet and stir everything for about 2 minutes.
7. Stir in the remaining ingredients except the cilantro and add more salt and pepper to taste.
8. Heat the stuffing for another 5 minutes until the ingredients are browned.
9. Turn off the heat, add dd the cilantro and divide the stuffing into the halved red bell peppers.
10. Put the peppers on a lightly greased baking tray and cover them with aluminum foil.
11. Place the tray in the oven for about 20 to 25 minutes.
12. Take the tray out and allow the bell peppers to sit for about 5 minutes.
13. Serve right away or allow the stuffed red bell peppers to cool down for storage!

STORAGE INFORMATION:

Storage	Temperature	Expiration date	Preparation
Ziploc bag	Fridge at 38 – 40°F or 3°C	3 days after preparation	Reheat in pot or microwave
Ziploc bag	Freezer at -1°F or -20°C	60 days after preparation	Thaw at room temperature. Reheat in pot or microwave

Note: The baked red bell peppers can be stored wrapped inside the aluminum foil used in the oven. Make sure the peppers have cooled before transferring them to a Ziploc bag or container.

16. Mexican Casserole

Serves: 4 | Prepping Time: ~ 30 min |

Total number of Ingredients: 11

Nutrition Information
(per serving)
- Calories: 442 kcal.
- Carbs: 65.9g.
- Fat: 11.5g.
- Protein: 20.2g.
- Fiber: 33.9g.
- Sugar: 17.4g.

INGREDIENTS:

- 1 cup dry black beans
- 1 cup dry white beans
- 1 tsp. olive oil
- 3 tbsp. Mexican spice (page 204)
- 2 cups Mexican salsa (page 49)
- 1½ cups cashew cheese spread (page 52)
- 3 bell peppers (red and yellow, chopped)
- 1 red onion (chopped)
- 1 green onion (chopped)
- 1 jalapeno pepper (medium, seeded and chopped)
- Salt and pepper to taste

METHOD

1. Cook the beans according to the recipe.
2. Preheat oven at 350°F or 175°C.
3. Grease a saucepan with the olive oil. Add Mexican spice, 1 cup of Mexican salsa and stir well.
4. Stir in the cashew cheese, chopped bell peppers, onions and add salt and pepper to taste.
5. Spread ½ cup salsa over the bottom of a casserole dish. Add the beans on top of the salsa and spread out the saucepan mix evenly over the beans.
6. Add the last ½ cup salsa sauce on top and sprinkle some chopped jalapenos on top.
7. Bake the casserole for 15-20 minutes.
8. Enjoy the dish after a short cooling period or let it cool down completely for storing.

STORAGE INFORMATION:

Storage	Temperature	Expiration date	Preparation
Airtight container M/L	Fridge at 38 – 40°F or 3°C	3-4 days after preparation	Reheat in microwave
Airtight container M/L	Freezer at -1°F or -20°C	60 days after preparation	Thaw at room temperature. Reheat in microwave

17. Quick Quinoa Casserole

Serves: 9 | Prep Time: ~15 min|

Total number of Ingredients: 17

Nutrition Information
(per serving)

- Calories: 236 kcal.
- Carbs: 24.9g.
- Fat: 11g.
- Protein: 9.2g.
- Fiber: 7.4g.
- Sugar: 4g.

INGREDIENTS:

- 2 cups dry pinto beans
- 1 cup dry quinoa
- 1 (7 oz.) pack tempeh (sliced)
- 2 tbsp. olive oil
- 2 tsp. cumin
- 2 tsp. paprika powder
- 1 cup red onion (diced)
- 2 garlic cloves (minced)
- 6 sweet red peppers (small, sliced)
- 2 (4 oz.) cans green chilies (diced)
- 1 cup Roma tomatoes (diced)
- 2 cups vegetable broth
- Salt and pepper to taste
- ½ cup no-salt cream cheese (page 61)
- 1 avocado (diced, sliced or mashed)
- ¼ cup green onions (diced)
- ¼ cup cilantro (chopped, fresh)

METHOD

1. Cook the pinto beans according to the recipe.
2. Put a large skillet greased with the olive oil over medium heat.
3. Grill the tempeh slices with a tsp. paprika powder, cumin and salt and pepper to taste for about 5 minutes.
4. Take out the grilled tempeh slices and leave it aside.
5. Grease the same skillet with olive oil and sauté the onions.
6. Add the minced garlic while stirring.
7. Blend in the red peppers and stir the ingredients for about 2 minutes.
8. Continue to add the green chilies, cooked pinto beans and quinoa, tomatoes and vegetable broth to the pan along with another tsp. of paprika powder, cumin, salt and pepper to taste.
9. Let the mixture cook for about 5 minutes.
10. Add the tempeh back to the skillet, stir, cover and reduce the heat to low.
11. Cook the mixture for about 15 minutes until the quinoa is soft and most of the broth has been absorbed.
12. Remove the skillet from the heat and add vegan cream cheese.
13. Put the lid on the skillet and let the dish sit for a minute until the cheese has melted.
14. Serve the quick quinoa casserole with fresh avocado slices, green onions and fresh cilantro.
15. Enjoy or store!

STORAGE INFORMATION:

Storage	Temperature	Expiration date	Preparation
Airtight container M/L	Fridge at 38 – 40°F or 3°C	3-4 days after preparation	Reheat in pot or microwave
Airtight container M/L	Freezer at -1°F or -20°C	60 days after preparation	Thaw at room temperature. Reheat in pot or microwave

18. Quinoa Greens Casserole

Serves: 5 | Prep Time: ~15 min |

Total number of Ingredients: 15

Nutrition Information
(per serving)
- Calories: 274 kcal.
- Carbs: 27g.
- Fat: 14.6g.
- Protein: 8.9g.
- Fiber: 3.3g.
- Sugar: 5.5g.

INGREDIENTS:

- 1½ cups dry quinoa
- 1½ cups broccoli florets (fresh or frozen)
- ½ cup panko
- 2 green onions (medium, chopped)
- 1 yellow onion (medium, chopped)
- 1 tsp. cornstarch
- 2 tbsp. avocado pesto (page 65)
- 2 tbsp. flour
- 2 cups vegetable broth (page 63)
- 2 tbsp. olive oil
- Salt and white pepper to taste
- 2 cups spinach
- ½ cup almond milk
- 1 cup cashew cheese spread (page 52)
- Handful fresh cilantro (optional)

METHOD

1. Preheat the oven to 375°F or 190°C.
2. Prepare the quinoa according to the recipe.
3. Steam the broccoli florets in a large sieve above the quinoa or in another pot with a small layer of boiling water for about 5 minutes.
4. Use a large baking dish, cover it with baking paper and put in the quinoa, broccoli, panko and onions.
5. Fill a medium-sized pot with water and put it on high heat.
6. Mix the cornstarch, flour, pesto, vegetable broth, olive oil, pepper and salt with the water in this pot and bring the mixture to a boil.
7. Once boiling, take the pot off and transfer the liquid to the large baking dish.
8. Add the spinach, almond milk and vegan cheese to the baking dish and stir thoroughly.
9. Bake the casserole for about 30 minutes in the oven.
10. Stir the casserole up with a wooden spoon and put it back in the oven for another 5-10 minutes.
11. Serve with white pepper and optional fresh cilantro on top.
12. Serve and enjoy, share or store in a container!

STORAGE INFORMATION:

Storage	Temperature	Expiration date	Preparation
Airtight container M/L	Fridge at 38 – 40°F or 3°C	2-3 days after preparation	Reheat in microwave
Airtight container M/L	Freezer at -1°F or -20°C	60 days after preparation	Thaw at room temperature. Reheat in microwave

19. Cashew Spaghetti with Asparagus

Serves: 4 | Prep Time: ~20 min |

Total number of Ingredients: 17

Nutrition Information
(per serving)
- Calories: 495 kcal.
- Carbs: 53.7g.
- Fat: 23.6g.
- Protein: 17g.
- Fiber: 11g.
- Sugar: 7g.

INGREDIENTS:

- 1 lb. whole-wheat spaghetti
- 5 tsp. olive oil
- 1 onion (large, chopped)
- 6 cloves garlic (chopped)
- 1 cup cashews (raw)
- 1 cup hot water
- 1 tbsp. tahini
- 1 lemon (medium, juiced)
- 1 tbsp. Dijon mustard
- 1 tbsp. nutritional yeast
- ½ tbsp. smoked paprika powder
- ½ tbsp. sweet paprika powder
- ¼ tsp. nutmeg
- 1 cup almond milk (unsweetened)
- 2 cups asparagus (chopped)
- ½ cup peas
- Salt and pepper to taste

METHOD

1. Fill a large pot with water, add some salt and bring it to a boil.
2. Cook the whole-wheat spaghetti according to the instructions or for 10-14 minutes.
3. In the meantime, take a medium skillet and add 3 tablespoons olive oil.
4. Put the skillet on medium heat and fry the onions and garlic until softened.
5. Blend the raw cashews with hot water in a blender for about 5 minutes.
6. Add the sautéed garlic, onion, tahini, lemon juice, Dijon mustard, yeast, paprika powders, nutmeg, salt and pepper to the blender.
7. Blend all these ingredients until the mixture has the consistency of a sauce.
8. Transfer the sauce to the previously used skillet and put it on medium heat.
9. Add the almond milk to the sauce and stir until the creamy substance has the desired thickness.
10. Drain the pasta and set it aside.
11. Fill up the pot with fresh water and bring to a boil.
12. Cook the chopped asparagus and peas with the remaining 2 tablespoons olive oil.
13. Drain the water from the pot after the vegetables are cooked.
14. Add the cooked spaghetti back in and stir well.
15. Pour the creamy sauce on top when serving.
16. Mix well and add more spices, salt or pepper to taste.
17. Enjoy!

STORAGE INFORMATION:

Storage	Temperature	Expiration date	Preparation
Airtight container L	Fridge at 38 – 40°F or 3°C	4-5 days after preparation	Reheat in pot or microwave
Airtight container L	Freezer at -1°F or -20°C	60 days after preparation	Thaw at room temperature. Reheat in pot or microwave

SNACKS & DESSERTS

1. Oatmeal Bars

Serves: 12 | Prep Time: ~10 min |

Total number of Ingredients: 14

Nutrition Information
(per serving)

- Calories: 455 kcal.
- Carbs: 36.1g.
- Fat: 31.1g.
- Protein: 9.6g.
- Fiber: 9g.
- Sugar: 18.2g.

INGREDIENTS:

- 1 cup dry red split lentils
- 1½ cups coconut flour
- 1 cup rolled oats
- 1 cup coconut flakes
  (unsweetened)
- 1 cup hemp seeds
- 2 tbsp. chia seeds
- 1 tsp. cinnamon
- 1 tsp. salt
- 1 cup dried blueberries
- 8 bananas (medium, ripe)
- 1 cup almond milk
- 1 cup coconut oil (melted)
- 1 tsp. vanilla extract
- 3 drops stevia sweetener

METHOD

1. Soak and drain the lentils according to the method. Dry the soaked lentils before using them in this dish.
2. Heat the oven to 350°F or 175°C.
3. Soak the chia seeds in water for about 15-30 minutes. Drain afterwards.
4. Line a baking tray with parchment paper and set it aside.
5. Mix together the coconut flour, oats, lentils, coconut flakes, hemp seeds, chia seeds, cinnamon, salt and blueberries in a large bowl and set it aside.
6. Mash the bananas in medium bowl and blend in the almond milk, coconut oil, vanilla extract and stevia.
7. Mix the ingredients in the medium bowl well. Then pour the wet mixture into the larger bowl.
8. Combine both mixtures with a mixer into a dough-like substance.
9. Use a spatula or your wet hands to evenly spread out the oat mixture in bar forms on the baking tray.
10. Place the tray in the oven for about 25 minutes, until edges of the bars are golden.
11. Take the tray out and let the bars cool down completely.
12. Optionally cut the bars into a smaller number of bars.
13. Serve and enjoy, share or wrap in foil and store for later!

STORAGE INFORMATION:

Storage	Temperature	Expiration date	Preparation
Wrapping foil or airtight container L	Fridge at 38 – 40°F or 3°C	5 days after preparation	
Wrapping foil or airtight container L	Freezer at -1°F or -20°C	60 days after preparation	Thaw at room temperature.

2. Breakfast Protein Bars

Serves: 16 | Prep Time: ~35 min |

Total number of Ingredients: 7

Nutrition Information
(per serving)

- Calories: 61 kcal.
- Carbs: 2.6g.
- Fat: 4.3g.
- Protein: 3.8g.
- Fiber: 1.3g.
- Sugar: 0.8g.

INGREDIENTS:

- 2 tbsp. cocoa butter
- 1 cup cashew cheese spread (page 52)
- 1 tsp. vanilla extract
- ¼ tsp. stevia
- ½ cup full-fat coconut milk
- 4 tbsp. coconut flour
- 2 scoops vegan protein powder

METHOD

1. Preheat the oven to 375°F or 190°C.
2. Whisk together the cocoa butter, cashew cheese spread, vanilla extract, stevia and coconut milk in a medium bowl until all the ingredients are completely mixed.
3. Stir in the coconut flour and protein powder. Mix again.
4. Pour the mixture into a baking sheet lined with parchment paper.
5. Transfer the sheet to the oven and bake the bars for about 15 minutes, until the batter has set.
6. Take out the baking sheet and let the bar chunk cool down.
7. Slice up the chunk into 16 bars.
8. Share and enjoy or wrap each bar in foil and store for another day!

STORAGE INFORMATION:

Storage	Temperature	Expiration date	Preparation
Airtight container M/L	Fridge at 38 – 40°F or 3°C	3-4 days after preparation	
Airtight container M/L	Freezer at -1°F or -20°C	60 days after preparation	Thaw at room temperature.

Note: Wrap each bar in wrapping foil makes storage and transport easier. It also helps to maintain taste and prevents dehydration.

3. Trail-Mix Energy Bars

Serves: 12 | Prep Time: ~25 min |

Total number of Ingredients: 10

Nutrition Information
(per serving)

- Calories: 302 kcal.
- Carbs: 44.9g.
- Fat: 10.4g.
- Protein: 7.2g.
- Fiber: 4.9g.
- Sugar: 22.6g.

INGREDIENTS:

- 2 cups rolled oats
- 2 cups puffed brown rice (page 53)
- 1 cup almonds (unsalted, chopped)
- ¼ cup roasted pumpkin seeds (unsalted)
- ¼ cup hemp seeds
- Pinch of salt
- 2 cups dates (pitted)
- ½ cup agave nectar (or maple syrup)
- ¼ cup sweet cashew cheese spread (page 46)
- 1 tbsp. vanilla extract

METHOD

1. Combine the oats, puffed rice, almonds, seeds and salt in a large bowl.
2. Blend the dates in a food processor, pulse until finely chopped.
3. Add the chopped dates to the dry ingredients and stir.
4. Take a small saucepan and put it on low heat.
5. Combine the agave nectar and cashew cheese spread in the pan. Prevent cooking it.
6. Use a mixer to combine the heated agave and cashew mixture with the dry ingredients.
7. Mix until smooth and creamy while adding the vanilla extract.
8. Line a bread form with parchment paper and pour the mixture down into this form.
9. Store the mix in the fridge for about 1 hour, until the batter has become hard.
10. Separate the chunk into 12 or 24 bars.
11. Enjoy or store wrapped in wrapping foil.

STORAGE INFORMATION:

Storage	Temperature	Expiration date	Preparation
Airtight container L or Ziploc bag	Fridge at 38 – 40°F or 3°C	3-4 days after preparation	
Airtight container L or Ziploc bag	Freezer at -1°F or -20°C	60 days after preparation	Thaw at room temperature.

4. No-Bake Nutella Bars

Serves: 8 | Prep Time: ~30 min |

Total number of Ingredients: 5

Nutrition Information
(per serving)
- Calories: 209 kcal.
- Carbs: 12.7g.
- Fat: 14.6g.
- Protein: 6.9g.
- Fiber: 3.9g.
- Sugar: 3.5g.

INGREDIENTS:
- 2 cups puffed brown rice (page 53)
- 1 cup chocolate hazelnut spread (page 55)
- 3 tbsp. vegan protein powder (vanilla or chocolate flavor)
- 9 drops stevia sweetener
- ¼ cup dark vegan chocolate (alternatively use ¼ cup cacao powder)

METHOD
1. Add the puffed rice, chocolate hazelnut spread, protein powder, stevia sweetener and chocolate to a large bowl.
2. Mix the ingredients together until the mixture has a thick and sticky consistency.
3. Line a bread form with parchment paper, pour the mixture in and press it down with a spatula or wooden spoon until it is packed in the bread form.
4. Place the bread form with the bar mixture in the freezer for 15 to 30 minutes, until the chunk is firm.
5. Take the form out of the freezer and remove the parchment paper. Cut the chunk into bars
6. Enjoy a bar alone or together. Store the others.

STORAGE INFORMATION:

Storage	Temperature	Expiration date	Preparation
Wrapping foil or airtight container L	Fridge at 38 – 40°F or 3°C	4-5 days after preparation	
Wrapping foil or airtight container L	Freezer at -1°F or -20°C	60 days after preparation	Thaw at room temperature.

5. Blueberry Almond Bites

Serves: 12 | Prep Time: ~35 min |

Total number of Ingredients: 8

Nutrition Information
(per serving)
- Calories: 226 kcal.
- Carbs: 6.1g.
- Fat: 17.2g.
- Protein: 12.5g.
- Fiber: 2.4g.
- Sugar: 2.5g.

INGREDIENTS:
- 1 cup peanut butter
- 2 tbsp. softened coconut butter
- ¼ tsp. stevia
- ½ cup full-fat coconut milk
- 4 tbsp. almond flour
- ¼ cup chopped almonds
- 2 tbsp. freeze-dried blueberry powder
- 2 scoops vegan protein powder

METHOD
1. Preheat the oven to 375°F or 190°C.
2. Grease a muffin tray with coconut oil.
3. Whisk the peanut butter, coconut butter, stevia and coconut milk in a large bowl until everything is thoroughly mixed.
4. Stir in the almond flour, almond bits, blueberry powder and protein powder. Mix well.
5. Pour the mixture into the muffin tray and make sure that each form is almost filled. Leave some space for the muffins to expand in the oven.
6. Bake the muffins for 10 minutes. Then turn the heat down to 350°F or 175°C.
7. Leave the muffins in the oven for another 5-10 minutes, until the batter has set.
8. Take out the muffin tray and let the muffins cool.
9. Store or enjoy!

STORAGE INFORMATION:

Storage	Temperature	Expiration date	Preparation
Airtight container L	Fridge at 38 – 40°F or 3°C	3-4 days after preparation	
Airtight container L	Freezer at -1°F or -20°C	60 days after preparation	Thaw at room temperature.

6. Mexikale Crisps

Total number of Ingredients: 9

Nutrition Information
(per serving)
- Calories: 313 kcal.
- Carbs: 33.4g.
- Fat: 14.6g.
- Protein: 12g.
- Fiber: 7g.
- Sugar: 0.3g.

INGREDIENTS:
- 8 cups kale leaves (large, chopped)
- 2 tbsp. avocado oil
- 2 tbsp. nutritional yeast
- 1 tsp. garlic powder
- 1 tsp. ground cumin
- ½ tsp. chili powder
- 1 tsp. dried oregano
- 1 tsp. dried cilantro
- Salt and pepper to taste

METHOD
1. Preheat the oven to 350°F or 175°C.
2. Line a baking tray with parchment paper and set it aside.
3. Absorb any remaining water from the chopped kale leaves with paper towels.
4. Place the chopped leaves in a large bowl and add the avocado oil, yeast and seasonings.
5. Mix and shake well before adding more yeast and extra seasonings if desired. Mix all the ingredients again.
6. Spread out the kale chips on the baking tray.
7. Bake the kale in the oven for 10-15 minutes. Check every minute after the 10-minute mark until the preferred crispiness is reached.
8. Take the tray out of the oven and set it aside to cool down.
9. Serve and enjoy or store in a container for later!

STORAGE INFORMATION:

Storage	Temperature	Expiration date	Preparation
Airtight container M	Fridge at 38 – 40°F or 3°C	4-5 days after preparation	
Airtight container M	Freezer at -1°F or -20°C	60 days after preparation	Thaw at room temperature.

7. Flaxseed Yogurt

Total number of Ingredients: 7

Nutrition Information
(per serving)
- Calories: 220 kcal.
- Carbs: 9.2g
- Fat: 16.9g
- Protein: 10g
- Fiber: 7.4g
- Sugar: 0.7g

INGREDIENTS:
- 2 cups water
- ½ cup hemp seeds
- ½ cup flax seeds
- 1 cup almond milk
- 2 tsp. psyllium husk
- ¼ cup lemon juice
- ¼ tsp. stevia

METHOD
1. Soak the flax seeds according the recipe. Drain the water.
2. Add 1 cup of boiling water to a heat resistant blender.
3. Continue to add the dry and soaked seeds.
4. Blend the ingredients for about 4 minutes.
5. Pour another cup of water, the almond milk and psyllium husk in the blender. Blend the mix again for 30 seconds.
6. Finally, add the lemon juice and stevia. Blend for another few seconds.
7. Pour the flaxseed yogurt into a container and put it in the fridge.
8. Serve the flaxseed yogurt chilled and enjoy or divide the yogurt for storing.

STORAGE INFORMATION:

Storage	Temperature	Expiration date	Preparation
Airtight container M	Fridge at 38 – 40°F or 3°C	3-4 days after preparation	
Airtight container M	Freezer at -1°F or -20°C	60 days after preparation	Thaw in fridge.

Note: The ingredients listed are good to produce 4 portions. Divide the yogurt over 4 airtight containers to serve or store the yogurt in portion sizes.

8. Raspberry Lemon Ice-Cream

Serves: 5 | Prep Time: ~90 min |

Total number of Ingredients: 6

Nutrition Information
(per serving)
- Calories: 198 kcal.
- Carbs: 8.3g
- Fat: 17.5g
- Protein: 1.8g
- Fiber: 3.9g
- Sugar: 4.0g

INGREDIENTS:

- 1 cup water
- 1 tsp. psyllium husk
- 1 lemon with peel
- 1 can full-fat coconut milk
- Pinch of stevia
- 1 cup raspberries

METHOD

1. Combine 1 cup of water with the psyllium husk in small pan over medium heat.
2. Stir thoroughly until the psyllium husk and water form a gel-like consistency.
3. Take about 1 tablespoon of lemon zest from the fresh lemon.
4. Combine the coconut milk, stevia, raspberries, tablespoon of lemon zest and all the lemon juice of the lemon with the psyllium husk mixture in a blender.
5. Blend the ingredients for about 3 minutes, until desired consistency is reached.
6. Transfer the mixture to a bowl. Transfer this bowl to the fridge and chill it for 1 hour.
7. Pour the mix into an ice-cream maker. Alternatively, pour all but ½ cup of the blended mixture into an ice cube tray and freeze it. After this part of the mixture is frozen, blend the cubes of mixture with the ½ cup unfrozen mixture to create delicious ice-cream.
8. Enjoy right away and/or store the ice cream in a container!

STORAGE INFORMATION:

Storage	Temperature	Expiration date	Preparation
Airtight container S	Freezer at -1°F or -20°C	60 days after preparation	Thaw slightly in the fridge.

9. Peanut Butter Brownies

Serves: 8 | Prep Time: ~15 min |

Total number of Ingredients: 7

Nutrition Information
(per serving)
- Calories: 142 kcal.
- Carbs: 6g.
- Fat: 8.8g.
- Protein: 10.2g.
- Fiber: 2.7g.
- Sugar: 1.9g.

INGREDIENTS:
- 1½ cups water
- ½ cup peanut butter
- 6 drops stevia
- ¼ cup cocoa powder
- 2 tsp. baking powder
- 2 scoops chocolate vegan protein powder (or flavor of choice)
- 2 tbsp. coconut flour
- ¼ cup almonds (optional)

METHOD
1. Preheat the oven to 350°F or 175°C.
2. Take a medium bowl and mix the lukewarm water, stevia and peanut butter into a smooth mixture.
3. Take another medium bowl and mix the cocoa powder, baking powder, vegan protein powder and coconut flour. Mix the ingredients well to avoid any remaining lumps.
4. Add the first mixture to the second mixture and combine both into a batter.
5. Pour the batter into a slightly greased oven dish, optionally lined with parchment paper.
6. Let the mixture bake for 40-45 minutes, until a knife comes out of the center clean.
7. Take out the oven dish and allow the brownie chunk to cool down before cutting it into 8 brownies.
8. Enjoy, share or store!

STORAGE INFORMATION:

Storage	Temperature	Expiration date	Preparation
Airtight container M	Fridge at 38 – 40°F or 3°C	3-4 days after preparation	
Airtight container M	Freezer at -1°F or -20°C	60 days after preparation	Thaw at room temperature.

Tip: Top with with almonds for a nice and crunchy flavour combination!

10. Mini Choco-Coco Cups

Serves: 10 cups | Prep Time: ~35 min |

Total number of Ingredients: 6

Nutrition Information
(per serving)
- Calories: 39 kcal.
- Carbs: 7.9g.
- Fat: 3.7g.
- Protein: 5.8g.
- Fiber: 5.5g.
- Sugar: 1.4g.

INGREDIENTS:

Coconut-based bottom:
- ½ cup coconut butter
- ½ cup coconut oil
- ½ cup shredded coconut
- 12 drops of stevia
- 1 tbsp. vanilla extract

Chocolate-based top:
- Milk-free dark chocolate

METHOD

1. Line a mini-muffin pan with mini cupcake liners.
2. Place the coconut butter and coconut oil in a pan on low heat. Melt both while stirring.
3. Add the shredded coconut, stevia, vanilla and stir again.
4. Pour the mixture into the cupcake liners. Put these in the freezer for about 30 minutes, until the mixture is firm.
5. Melt the chocolate au bain-marie over medium-low heat. Scoop the molten chocolate over the hardened coconut cups.
6. Place the cups in the refrigerator. Keep them refrigerated for about an hour, until the cups are firm like candy.
7. Store or enjoy right away!

STORAGE INFORMATION:

Storage	Temperature	Expiration date	Preparation
Airtight container M	Fridge at 38 – 40°F or 3°C	3-4 days after preparation	
Airtight container M	Freezer at -1°F or -20°C	60 days after preparation	Thaw at room temperature.

Note: This combination paired with the chocolate on top is great for satisfying cravings and provides a quick energy boost.

11. Almond Cookies

Total number of Ingredients: 9

Nutrition Information
(per serving)

- Calories: 77 kcal.
- Carbs: 1.7g.
- Fat: 6.2g.
- Protein: 1.3g.
- Fiber: 0.9g.
- Sugar: 0.6g.

INGREDIENTS:

- 1 cup almond butter
- 1 tsp. vanilla extract
- ½ tsp. stevia
- ¾ cup almond flour
- 1 tsp. baking soda
- ¼ cup water

Filling:

- 2/3 cup almonds (crushed)
- 2 tbsp. coconut flour (alternatively use almond flour)
- ½ tsp. stevia
- 2 tbsp. water

METHOD

1. Preheat the oven to 350°F or 175°C.
2. Mix the almond butter, water, vanilla extract and stevia together in large bowl.
3. Stir in the almond flour and baking soda until all ingredients are completely mixed. Use a mixer if necessary or preferred.
4. Let the dough rest for a few minutes.
5. Combine the crushed almonds, coconut flour, stevia and 2 tablespoons of water in a small bowl and set it aside.
6. Roll the cookie dough from the first bowl out between two sheets of parchment paper in a ¼ inch thick square.
7. Remove the top parchment paper and add a layer of filling from the small bowl to the dough by spreading it around. Cover the square again, flip it around and repeat this process for the other side. Make sure to leave about ½ inch of uncovered space on the sides.
8. Carefully roll the cookie dough into a log on a piece of parchment paper. Use more paper to do so if necessary.
9. Chill the dough log in the freezer for 15-20 minutes, until firm.
10. Take the dough from the freezer and carefully remove the parchment paper.
11. Cut the log into 24 slices of about ½ inch thick.
12. Place the slices on a cookie sheet or baking plate lined with parchment paper. Make sure to leave enough space between each cookie. Bake in two batches if necessary.
13. Bake the cookies for 20-25 minutes, until the edges turn golden.
14. Remove the cookies from the oven and allow them to cool down for 30 minutes.
15. Bake the second batch, if necessary.
16. Enjoy, share or store the cookies!

STORAGE INFORMATION:

Storage	Temperature	Expiration date	Preparation
Airtight container L	Fridge at 38 – 40°F or 3°C	4-5 days after preparation	
Airtight container L	Freezer at -1°F or -20°C	60 days after preparation	Thaw at room temperature.

12. Banana & Blueberry Muffins

Serves: 12 | Prep Time: ~35 min |

Total number of Ingredients: 10

Nutrition Information
(per serving)

- Calories: 236 kcal.
- Carbs: 17.8g.
- Fat: 16.3g.
- Protein: 4.6g.
- Fiber: 3.8g.
- Sugar: 8.7g.

INGREDIENTS:

- 2 cups almond flour
- 1 tsp. baking soda
- ½ tsp. salt
- ¼ tsp. cinnamon
- 5 bananas (medium, ripe)
- ¼ cup coconut oil
- ½ cup almond milk
- 2 tsp. vanilla extract
- 1½ cup blueberries (fresh or frozen)

METHOD

1. Preheat the oven to 350°F or 175°C.
2. Place paper muffin liners in a muffin pan and set it aside.
3. Take a medium bowl and whisk the flour, baking powder, baking soda, salt and cinnamon.
4. Take another large bowl and mash the bananas in it.
5. Add the coconut oil, almond milk and vanilla extract to the banana bowl. Mix all the ingredients until all the ingredients in it are combined well.
6. Slowly stir the dry ingredients from the first bowl into the banana mix.
7. Mix thoroughly before carefully folding in the blueberries.
8. Spoon the mixture into the muffin liners until all are about three-quarters filled.
9. Bake the muffins for 20-25 minutes, until a knife stuck in the muffin comes out clean.
10. Take the muffins out of the oven and let them cool down completely before taking the muffin liners off.
11. Store for later or enjoy right away!

STORAGE INFORMATION:

Storage	Temperature	Expiration date	Preparation
Airtight container L	Fridge at 38 – 40°F or 3°C	4-5 days after preparation	
Airtight container L	Freezer at -1°F or -20°C	60 days after preparation	Thaw at room temperature.

Tip: Serve with crushed almonds on top vor a more crunchy bite!

13. Chai Latte

Serves: 8 | Prep Time: ~40 min |

Total number of Ingredients: 11

Nutrition Information
(per serving)
- Calories: 339 kcal.
- Carbs: 7.3g.
- Fat: 33.4g.
- Protein: 2.4g.
- Fiber: 2.9g.
- Sugar: 4.0g.

INGREDIENTS:
- ¼ cup cocoa butter
- 1 cup pre-made tea of your choice
  (lemon is recommended)
- 2 cups water
- 4 cups full-fat coconut milk
- ½ tsp. stevia
- 3 tsp. cinnamon
- 6 green cardamom pods (cracked)
- 6 cloves (whole)
- 6 black peppercorns
- 1 tbsp. minced ginger
- ¼ cup vegan half-and-half cream
  (optional, see page 56)

METHOD

1. Put the cocoa butter, tea, water, coconut milk, stevia, cinnamon, cloves, cardamom, peppercorns and ginger in a pan and bring it to a soft boil.
2. Once the mixture is boiling, lower the heat and allow the latte to softly simmer for 15-20 minutes, until the cocoa butter is fully dissolved.
3. Allow the mixture to cool, then strain it with a cheese cloth into a jar.
4. Pour a serving of the strained tea into a cup.
5. Heat the cup in the microwave and finally add the optional half-and-half cream.
6. Stir, serve and enjoy. Store the other tea in the jar.

STORAGE INFORMATION:

Storage	Temperature	Expiration date	Preparation
Airtight container M	Fridge at 38 – 40°F or 3°C	3-4 days after preparation	Reheat in pot or microwave
Airtight container M	Freezer at -1°F or -20°C	60 days after preparation	Thaw at room temperature. Reheat in pot or microwave

14. Maple Spelt Cookies

Total number of Ingredients: 11

Nutrition Information
(per serving)
 - Calories: 338 kcal.
 - Carbs: 42.4g.
 - Fat: 15.2g.
 - Protein: 8g.
 - Fiber: 5g.
 - Sugar: 20.3g.

INGREDIENTS:
 - 4 bananas (medium, ripe)
 - 5 cups spelt flour
 - Pinch of salt
 - 2 tsp. cinnamon
 - 2 cups sweet cashew cheese spread
   (page 46)
 - ½ cup almonds
 - ½ cup walnuts
 - ½ cup hazelnuts
 - 1½ cups dried fruits (of choice)
 - 2 tsp. vanilla extract
 - ½ cup maple syrup

METHOD
1. Preheat oven to 350°F or 175°C.
2. Line a baking sheet with parchment paper.
3. Mash the bananas in a large bowl.
4. Blend in the spelt flour, salt, cinnamon, cashew cheese, nuts, fruits, vanilla extract and maple syrup until a smooth dough has formed.
5. Use a tablespoon and drop a small dough ball onto the parchment paper.
6. Flatten the dough ball gently with the spoon. Repeat this process and keep 2-inches of space between the dough balls.
7. Place the tray with cookies in the oven for 20 minutes until golden brown.
8. Take the tray out of the oven and let the cookies cool down completely.
9. Store or enjoy right away!

STORAGE INFORMATION:

Storage	Temperature	Expiration date	Preparation
Airtight container M/L	Fridge at 38 – 40°F or 3°C	5-6 days after preparation	
Airtight container M/L	Freezer at -1°F or -20°C	60 days after preparation	Thaw at room temperature.

15. Peach-Cake Cheeseballs

Serves: 8 | Prep Time: ~20 min |

Total number of Ingredients: 6

Nutrition Information
(per serving)
- Calories: 182 kcal.
- Carbs: 8g.
- Fat: 10.8g.
- Protein: 13.1g.
- Fiber: 1.6g.
- Sugar: 4.3g.

INGREDIENTS:
- ½ cup coconut cream
- 2 tbsp. sweet cashew cheese spread (page 46)
- 3 scoops vegan protein powder
- ½ cup ground hemp seeds
- ¼ cup freeze dried peach powder
- 1 tsp. nutritional yeast

METHOD
1. Melt the coconut cream in a pan on low heat. Make sure the cream doesn't start boiling.
2. Mix in the hazelnut spread and stir well.
3. Take the pan off the heat and add the protein powder, ground hemp seeds, peach powder and nutritional yeast.
4. Mix all the ingredients thoroughly into a smooth dough.
5. Roll the dough into 16 balls.
6. Chill the balls for a few minutes before serving or storing!

STORAGE INFORMATION:

Storage	Temperature	Expiration date	Preparation
Airtight container M/L	Fridge at 38 – 40°F or 3°C	3-4 days after preparation	
Airtight container M/L	Freezer at -1°F or -20°C	60 days after preparation	Thaw at room temperature.

16. Pumpkin Oat Muffins

Serves: 20 | Prep Time: ~50 min |

Total number of Ingredients: 12

Nutrition Information
(per serving)
- Calories: 130 kcal.
- Carbs: 22.8g.
- Fat: 2.8g.
- Protein: 3.6g.
- Fiber: 3.5g.
- Sugar: 4.4g.

INGREDIENTS:
- 3 cups whole wheat flour
- 2 cups oatmeal
- 2 tsp. baking soda
- 4 tsp. pumpkin pie spice (page 204)
- ½ tsp. salt
- 2 bananas (medium, ripe)
- 1 cup pumpkin flesh
- 1½ cup almond milk (unsweetened)
- ¼ cup applesauce (page 51)
- 4 flax eggs (page 47)
- ½ cup dark chocolate chips (dairy-free)

METHOD
1. Heat the oven to 350°F or 175°C.
2. Line 12 baking cups in a cupcake tray.
3. Mix the flour, most of the oatmeal, baking soda, pumpkin spice and salt in a large bowl. Make sure to mix well.
4. Mash the bananas into another medium bowl, along with the pumpkin flesh, almond milk, apple sauce and flax eggs.
5. Mix both mixtures from each bowl together in the large bowl. Combine well.
6. Add the chocolate chips and mix again.
7. Fill each cupcake cup with a scoop of batter and sprinkle them with some additional oats on top.
8. Place the tray in the oven for about 25 minutes.
9. Take the tray out and allow the muffins to cool down before consumption or storage.

STORAGE INFORMATION:

Storage	Temperature	Expiration date	Preparation
Airtight container L	Fridge at 38 – 40°F or 3°C	5 days after preparation	
Airtight container L	Freezer at -1°F or -20°C	60 days after preparation	Thaw at room temperature.

17. Raspberry Cheesecake

Serves: 16 | Prep Time: ~10 min |

Total number of Ingredients: 9

Nutrition Information
(per serving)
- Calories: 262 kcal
- Carbs: 8.2g
- Fat: 23g
- Protein: 5.6g
- Fiber: 1.7g
- Sugar: 1.7g

INGREDIENTS:

Pie crust:
- 8 tbsp. hemp seeds
- 8 tbsp. finely shredded coconut
- 1 tsp. vanilla extract

Filling:
- 2 cups raw cashews
- 2 cups no-salt cream cheese (page 61)
- 1 cup raspberries (fresh or frozen)
- 4 tbsp. MCT oil
- 2 tbsp. lime juice
- ½ tsp. stevia

METHOD

1. Soak the cashews in water for 8 hours.
2. Mix the crust ingredients in a medium bowl.
3. Transfer the mixture and flatten it into a layer in a deep baking dish.
4. Drain the cashews and combine all the filling ingredients in blender until the cake filling is a smooth mixture. Scrape down the sides of the blender if necessary.
5. Add an even layer of filling over the crust.
6. Place the baking dish in the freezer for about 2 hours. Let the cheesecake chill until firm.
7. Serve the cake with some additional fresh or frozen raspberries on top.
8. Enjoy the cheesecake right away or store it in container(s) for later!

STORAGE INFORMATION:

Storage	Temperature	Expiration date	Preparation
Airtight container L	Fridge at 38 – 40°F or 3°C	3-4 days after preparation	
Airtight container L	Freezer at -1°F or -20°C	60 days after preparation	Thaw in fridge.

Tip: Serve with extra forest fruits and berries on top and garnish with powdered sugar for a delicious treat!

18. Mini Hazelnut Doughnuts

Serves: 24 | Prep Time: ~35 min |

Total number of Ingredients: 9

Nutrition Information
(per serving)
- Calories: 116 kcal.
- Carbs: 2.8g.
- Fat: 9.8g.
- Protein: 4.8g.
- Fiber: 2.4g.
- Sugar: 1.1g.

INGREDIENTS:

- 4 tbsp. ground hemp seeds
- 2 tbsp. MCT oil
- ½ cup water
- ¼ tsp. stevia
- 2 tbsp. flaxseed oil
- 1 tsp. vanilla extract
- 1 tsp. baking powder
- 2 cups almond flour
- ½ cup chocolate hazelnut spread
  (page 55)

METHOD

1. Preheat the oven to 350°F or 175°C.
2. Grease a muffin plate or a doughnut pan with MCT oil.
3. Combine the hemp seeds with the water in a medium bowl and stir.
4. Continue to stir in the stevia, flaxseed oil and vanilla extract.
5. Mix the baking powder with the flour in another medium bowl and set it aside.
6. Combine the chocolate hazelnut spread with the wet hemp seed mixture and stir thoroughly.
7. Mix the flour and baking powder with the wet mixture into a smooth dough.
8. Transfer scoops of the batter to the doughnut pan or muffin plate.
9. Put the pan or plate in the oven and bake the doughnuts for about 30 minutes.
10. Take the pan or tray out and allow the doughnuts to cool.
11. Enjoy, share or store!

STORAGE INFORMATION:

Storage	Temperature	Expiration date	Preparation
Airtight container L	Fridge at 38 – 40°F or 3°C	4-5 days after preparation	
Airtight container L	Freezer at -1°F or -20°C	60 days after preparation	Thaw at room temperature.

19. Tropical Chips

Serves: 2 | Prep Time: ~ 20 min |

Total number of Ingredients: 6

Nutrition Information
(per serving)
- Calories: 611 kcal.
- Carbs: 136.5g.
- Fat: 5g.
- Protein: 5g.
- Fiber: 16.4g.
- Sugar: 100.5g.

INGREDIENTS:

- 2 apples (thin slices, dehydrate for 8-10 hours)
- 1 pineapple (thin slices, dehydrate for 12-20 hours)
- 2 bananas (thin slices, dehydrate for 12-20 hours)
- 1 mango (thin slices, dehydrate for 12-20 hours)

Lemon-Water Solution:
- ½ cup lemon juice
- 1½ water

METHOD

1. Put the lemon juice and water in a spray bottle.
2. Start with the apple slices by laying them out on the dehydrator tray.
3. Make sure the slices do not overlap each other. The same goes for the other fruits.
4. Spray the top side of the fruit slices with the lemon water.
5. Spray and dehydrate the fruits in multiple batches.
6. Place trays in the dehydrator and set the temperature to 115-120 F.
7. When using a dehydrator with a timer, set it according to the times per fruit. In case fruits are combined, take the apple slices out first.
8. Dehydrate all the fruit slices. Keep an eye on the slices in the final hours.
9. Enjoy, incorporate in a salad or store!

STORAGE INFORMATION:

Storage	Temperature	Expiration date	Preparation
Airtight container M	Fridge at 38 – 40°F or 3°C	5 days after preparation	
Airtight container M	Freezer at -1°F or -20°C	60 days after preparation	Thaw at room temperature.

20. Sesame Seed Cheese

Serves: 1 bowl of cheese / 12 wedges | Prep Time: ~10 min |

Total number of Ingredients: 7

Nutrition Information (per wedge)

- Calories: 57 kcal.
- Carbs: 2.0g
- Fat: 4.9g
- Protein: 1.0g
- Fiber: 0.8g
- Sugar: 0g

INGREDIENTS:

- 1 tsp. nutritional yeast
- ½ cup sesame seeds
- 2 tbsp. olive oil
- ¼ tsp. salt
- 1 cup water
- 1 tbsp. agar-agar
- ¼ tsp. garlic powder

METHOD

1. Mix the nutritional yeast, sesame seeds, olive oil and salt in a medium bowl into a thick, sticky mixture.
2. Put a medium pot filled with 1 cup water on low heat.
3. Bring the water to a simmer and stir in the agar-agar.
4. Turn off heat and let the water cool for 5 minutes.
5. Blend the warm water with agar-agar, garlic powder and sesame seed mixture. Mix the ingredients well using a whisk or a mixer.
6. Pour the cheese mix into a large bowl and cover it with wrapping foil.
7. Refrigerate the cheese until firm.
8. Serve or store!

STORAGE INFORMATION:

Storage	Temperature	Expiration date	Preparation
Airtight container L	Fridge at 38 – 40°F or 3°C	3-4 days after preparation	
Airtight container L	Freezer at -1°F or -20°C	60 days after preparation	Thaw at room temperature.

21. Pumpkin Pie Bites

Serves: 15 | Prep Time: ~20 min |

Total number of Ingredients: 6

Nutrition Information
(per serving)
- Calories: 124 kcal.
- Carbs: 2.3g.
- Fat: 12.4g.
- Protein: 0.7g.
- Fiber: 2.0g.
- Sugar: 0.7g.

INGREDIENTS:
- ½ cup pumpkin puree
- ½ cup coconut oil
- ¼ cup coconut butter
- 3 drops stevia (or alternative vegan sweetener)
- 2 tsp. cinnamon
- ½ cup pecans

METHOD
1. Combine the pumpkin puree, coconut oil and coconut butter in a large bowl.
2. Stir in the stevia and cinnamon.
3. Mix the ingredients together evenly with a whisk or mixer.
4. Continue to transfer the mix into mini-molds or an ice cube tray.
5. Refrigerate the bites until firm, for about 1 hour.
6. Top the bites with the pecan nuts.
7. Serve, share or enjoy!

STORAGE INFORMATION:

Storage	Temperature	Expiration date	Preparation
Airtight container M	Fridge at 38 – 40°F or 3°C	4-5 days after preparation	
Airtight container M	Freezer at -1°F or -20°C	60 days after preparation	Thaw at room temperature.

Tip: A special for pumpkin lovers!

22. Walnut Chocolate Bites

Serves: 8 | Prep Time: ~15 min |

Total number of Ingredients: 5

Nutrition Information
(per serving)
- Calories: 185 kcal.
- Carbs: 4.5g.
- Fat: 17.9g.
- Protein: 1.7g.
- Fiber: 1.5g.
- Sugar: 2.5g.

INGREDIENTS:
- ½ cup coconut oil
- 4 tbsp. cocoa powder
- 1 tbsp. sugar (or vegan sweetener of choice)
- 2 tbsp. tahini paste
- ¼ cup halved walnuts

METHOD
1. Place a pot on low heat.
2. Add the coconut oil and stir until the oil is melted.
3. Add the cocoa powder, sugar and tahini. Make sure to mix everything thoroughly.
4. Let the mixture cool and pour it into molds or ice trays.
5. Place the molds or ice trays in the refrigerator for about 5-10 minutes.
6. Continue to add a halved walnut on top of each bite.
7. Refrigerate the bites for another 20 minutes.
8. Serve or store the bites once they are ready for consumption.

STORAGE INFORMATION:

Storage	Temperature	Expiration date	Preparation
Airtight container S	Fridge at 38 – 40°F or 3°C	3-4 days after preparation	
Airtight container S	Freezer at -1°F or -20°C	60 days after preparation	Thaw at room temperature.

How to use the included meal plan

Prepping your meals is a real game changer. As in many of life's pursuits, forming habits will yield the best results, so develop a routine right from the start. Pick one or two days per week when you can dedicate 2-4 hours to cooking. (Choose two days rather than one if you have limited storage space or smaller time windows per day.) Make sure to have all ingredients ready and prepare labels for each meal you're about to prep.

KEEP A SCHEDULE

Keeping a schedule in your agenda, notebook, or smartphone will help you remember what to eat at your predetermined dates and times. Label all prepped dishes according to this schedule. Write both the recipe name and the date you plan to eat it on the label and on your schedule. This will reduce confusion, and you can avoid consulting your meal plan each time you sit down to eat. Proper labeling and writing down your meals for the day will make it super easy to stick to your plan, reduce stress, and reach your fitness goals!

Following the meal plan strictly, for the full 30 days, can require you to prepare up to 25 recipes per week. But this is not necessary; the best way to follow the meal plan in this book is to pick one or two days with recipes you enjoy and prep these recipes for multiple days in row.

MACRONUTRIENTS AND DAILY CALORIE INTAKE

Each day of the meal plan guarantees a proper number of balanced macronutrients. Depending on your nutritional needs, you can determine the appropriate number of servings. Choose two or more daily sets of recipes that you can alternate throughout the week, so you can have variety while only needing to prepare four to eight recipes per prepping session. Following a meal plan doesn't have to be boring; you can change your preferences each week.

Each day in the included meal plan consists of five meals: breakfast, two snacks, lunch, and dinner. These meals may vary in serving size. The daily meal plan provides portions for 1600, 1800, 2000, 2500 or 3000 kcal per day. Depending on your bodyweight and goals, it's important to aim for a calorie deficit for weight loss, or a surplus of calories and macros for muscle growth.

Consuming one gram of protein per day for each lean pound of your body weight is recommended for gaining muscle. If your meals on a given day of the meal plan don't deliver enough protein, you can supplement with one or more protein shakes. Note that these shakes also have nutritional value, so this calorie amount should be included in the total daily calories. Always keep track of your macronutrient and calorie intake and physical results, but keep in mind that small changes won't affect your weight or progress right away.

If you want to make any changes to the meal plan, which is not recommended, it's important to stick to the given macro balances. If you want to replace one or more meals because you don't like them, recalculate the macro values and swap in equivalent meals from different days of the plan. A notepad will make it easy to recalculate macro values.

Tip: Use an app, Excel sheet, or a notepad to keep track of your macro intake. This will save you headaches and guarantee the right number of macros for every day of the week. Some great apps include MyMacros+, MyFitnessPal and Nutritionist.

Ultimately, the goal is to find a meal prepping routine that works for you. Cook on days that you prefer, but always plan ahead of time to prevent an empty fridge or freezer. You have the flexibility to interchange days of the meal plan but stick to the prescribed portion sizes and macro amounts, and keep track of your macronutrient and calorie intake.

Make meal prepping a habitual part of your lifestyle and you'll find it a lot easier to reach your health and fitness goals!

CREATING A MATCHING SHOPPING LIST AND GROCERY SHOPPING

Create a shopping list to optimize each trip to the grocery store. First, make sure to list all the ingredients required for the recipes you plan to prepare in your upcoming prepping session(s). Remember that you can choose to prep either once or twice per week. You can buy all the ingredients for the entire week in a single grocery shopping session but do consider the expiration date of ingredients. You might want to buy fresh ingredients with a limited shelf life more often than once a week.

Another thing to consider is your pantry. A seasoned meal prepper keeps his or her pantry stocked with nonperishables and keeps track of what is running low or nearing expiration.

Make sure that on each trip to the grocery store (or stores, if you buy your ingredients in different places), you bring a list and stick to it. Preparing a complete list will ensure that you have all the ingredients required when it's time to cook the dishes on prepping days. Buying only what's necessary will help you save money and prevent waste.

Save your lists to a cloud storage service like Google Drive so you can access them anytime and anywhere with your smartphone. This way, you'll always be able to access it during your shopping trip. Alternatively, you can sign up for a grocery delivery service like Amazon Prime or Instacart. These apps enable you to save your list in the app and have all your groceries delivered before you start cooking for the next week of meal prep!

Note: Shopping lists for each week of the complete 30-day meal plan can be found at: http://happyhealthygreen.life/meal-prep/shopping-lists

Prepping and Storing Food

The freezer is one of the most useful devices when meal prepping but to make life easier, there are some things to keep in mind. It is a good idea to regularly clean out your freezer. Store your food at room temperature or in the refrigerator before freezing so that your food is not hot when you put it in- which thaws the ice and food around it.

Keeping the freezer full is more economical and air will be kept cold more easily but don't overload it so that no air can circulate. Be careful not to keep the door open for long when taking food in and out as the food inside will start to defrost and go bad.

Vegan ingredients that are easy to prepare

VEGETABLES AND BEANS

Blanch your beans and vegetables before freezing them to preserve their color, texture and flavor. Cooked vegetable purees and beans can also go into the freezer. The blanching process is explained below.

FRUIT

Frozen fruits are great for smoothies. Fruits that freeze well include apples, olives, avocados, pears, kiwis, oranges, grapefruit, lemons, limes, peaches, plums, nectarines, bananas, raspberries, blackberries, watermelon, honeydew melons, cantaloupe, apricots, grapes, mangoes, cherries, strawberries, blueberries, raisins, currants, cranberries, dates and figs.

OTHER VEGAN FOODS THAT CAN BE FROZEN

Seeds that can be frozen include: almonds, cashews, walnuts, pecans, sunflower seeds, sunflower seed butter, pumpkin seeds, chia seeds, ground flaxseed and sesame seeds.

Herbs and spices such as oregano, thyme, cumin, turmeric, chili powder, cinnamon, pepper, salsa, soy sauce and mustard are also freezer-friendly. To freeze herbs, remove the leaves from the stems and allow the herbs to dry by leaving them out in the air. After drying, place the herbs in a bag and into the freezer.

Grains, beans and legumes also freeze well. Vegetables like peas, runner, French, dwarf and broad beans, asparagus and broccoli can go into the freezer as well.

WHAT NOT TO FREEZE

Vegetables high in water content, including cucumber, lettuce, bean sprouts, cauliflower florets, zucchini and tomatoes do not freeze well and must be blanched first. If they are not blanched, they become limp or mushy when thawed. Herbs like basil, chives and parsley will suffer from freezer burn. Carrots will become rubbery if frozen and potatoes, unless they are cooked first, will undergo texture change.

WHAT IS BLANCHING?

Blanching involves rapid heating and cooling to remove moisture from a vegetable. Vegetables are placed in a blanching pot basket surrounded by boiling water. After 2 minutes, the basket is removed and quickly transferred to a tub of cold water before being drained. Vegetables are then ready to put in the freezer.

Perfecting the art of prepping

BENEFITS OF LONG-TERM MEAL PREPPING

Once you get into the rhythm of vegan meal prepping, stress relief will follow. Having meals prepared in advance means no last-minute rush to prepare or buy a meal just in time to eat; particularly after work, when you are already tired and would rather engage in other activities.

Meal prepping is a wonderful investment for your health, both mental and physical. You will be relieved of daily decisions and meal preparation fatigue, you will lose weight or get in shape and are likely to see improvements in your cardiovascular health.

BECOMING AN AMAZING COOK

Being able to cook and prepare great meals is extremely rewarding and is a skill that can be learned.

You will learn to tackle food waste as you learn to manage ingredients and turn leftovers into another delicious meal. For example, leftover broccoli can be incorporated in salads, soups, curries and rice dishes.

In the long-term, meal prepping will aid you in balancing other areas of your life—your fridge will be neater, your kitchen cleaner and you will free up more time for other important activities.

The 30-Day Vegan Meal Plan

Week 1: Meal Plan

MEAL PLAN	MONDAY	
BREAKFAST	*GARDEN GREEN SMOOTHIE*	1/2 Serving
A.M. SNACK	*MAPLE SPELT COOKIES*	1 Serving
LUNCH	*CHICKPEA COUSCOUS*	2 Servings
P.M. SNACK	*RASPBERRY LEMON ICE CREAM*	1 Serving
DINNER	*TRIPLE BEAN CHILI*	2 Servings
TOTAL		

FAT	CARBS	PROTEIN	CALORIES	SERVINGS	SERVINGS	SERVINGS	SERVINGS
12	25,2	14	265	1/2	1/2	1/2	1
15,2	42,4	8	338	1	1	2	2
12	88,4	20	540	2	2	2	3
17,5	8,3	1,8	198	2	3	3	3
7	46	11,8	286	2	2	3	3
63,7 gr.	**210,3 gr.**	**55,6 gr.**	1627 kcal.	1825 kcal.	2023 kcal.	2504 kcal.	3039 kcal.

MEAL PLAN	TUESDAY	
BREAKFAST	*PEACHY MANGO BOWL*	1/2 Serving
A.M. SNACK	*OATMEAL BARS*	1/2 Serving
LUNCH	*SWEET POTATO CHICKPEA MINGLE*	1 Serving
P.M. SNACK	*MINI HAZELNUT DOUGHNUTS*	1 Serving
DINNER	*TEMPEH CURRY*	1 Serving
TOTAL		

FAT	CARBS	PROTEIN	CALORIES	SERVINGS	SERVINGS	SERVINGS	SERVINGS
24,9	49	7,7	451	1/2	1/2	1/2	1/2
15,5	18	4,8	227	1	1	1	1
20,2	33,4	16	379	1	1	1	2
9,8	2,8	4,8	116	1	3	3	4
13,75	44,5	27,5	411	1	1	2	2
84,15 gr.	147,7 gr.	60,8 gr.	1584 kcal.	1811 kcal.	2043 kcal.	2454 kcal.	2949kcal.

MEAL PLAN	WEDNESDAY	
BREAKFAST	*GARDEN GREEN SMOOTHIE*	1/2 Serving
A.M. SNACK	*MINI HAZELNUT DOUGHNUTS*	1 Serving
LUNCH	*VEGAN GOULASH*	1 Serving
P.M. SNACK	*MANGO BLASTER SMOOTHIE*	1 Serving
DINNER	*QUINOA AND BROCCOLI STEW*	1 Serving
TOTAL		

FAT	CARBS	PROTEIN	CALORIES	SERVINGS	SERVINGS	SERVINGS	SERVINGS
12	25,2	14	265	1/2	1/2	1/2	1/2
9,8	2,8	4,8	116	1	3	4	6
18,7	83,8	16,5	591	1	1	1	1
8,2	61	3,4	331	1/2	1/2	1	1
10	47	12	326	1	1	1	2
58,7 gr.	219,8 gr.	50,7 gr.	1629 kcal.	1795 kcal.	2027 kcal.	2474 kcal.	3032 kcal.

MEAL PLAN		THURSDAY	
BREAKFAST	BERRY GREEN SMOOTHIE BAG		1/2 Serving
A.M. SNACK	FLAXSEED YOGURT		1 Serving
LUNCH	BLACK BEAN BURGERS		2 Servings
P.M. SNACK	MINI CHOCO-COCO CUPS		3 Servings
DINNER	GOLDEN TOFU NOODLE BOWL		1/2 Serving
TOTAL			

FAT	CARBS	PROTEIN	CALORIES	SERVINGS	SERVINGS	SERVINGS	SERVINGS
26	54	6	472	1/2	1/2	1/2	1/2
16,9	9,2	10	220	1	2	3	3
3,2	36,2	19,8	414	3	3	3	5
11,1	23,7	17,4	264	5	5	5	6
11,2	31,6	11,7	273	1/2	1/2	1	1
68,4 gr.	154,7 gr.	64,9 gr.	1643 kcal.	1819 kcal.	2039 kcal.	2532 kcal.	3034 kcal.

MEAL PLAN		FRIDAY	
BREAKFAST	GARDEN GREEN SMOOTHIE		1/2 Servings
A.M. SNACK	BREAKFAST PROTEIN BARS		2 Servings
LUNCH	RISOTTO		1 Serving
P.M. SNACK	FLAXSEED YOGURT		1 Serving
DINNER	BROCCOLI QUICHE		1 Serving
TOTAL			

FAT	CARBS	PROTEIN	CALORIES	SERVINGS	SERVINGS	SERVINGS	SERVINGS
24	50,5	28	530	1	1	1	1
8,6	5,2	7,6	122	4	4	6	8
22,1	43,6	8,3	406	1	1	1	2
16,9	9,2	10	220	1	2	2	2
19	43,1	8,8	378	1	1	2	2
90,6 gr.	151,6 gr.	62,7 gr.	1656 kcal.	1780 kcal.	1992 kcal.	2488 kcal.	3016 kcal.

Week 2: Meal Plan

MEAL PLAN	MONDAY	
BRAEKFAST	*BREAKFAST OATS BOWL*	2/3 Servings
A.M. SNACK	*PUMPKIN OAT MUFFINS*	1 Serving
LUNCH	*BLACK BEAN BURGERS*	2 Servings
P.M. SNACK	*NO-BAKE NUTELLA BARS*	1 Serving
DINNER	*TEMPEH CURRY*	1 Serving
TOTAL		

FAT	CARBS	PROTEIN	CALORIES	SERVINGS	SERVINGS	SERVINGS	SERVINGS
19,6	50,8	9	415	1	1	1	1
2,8	22,8	3,6	130	1	1	2	3
6,4	72,4	19,8	426	2	3	3	4
14,6	12,7	6,9	209	1	1	1	2
13,7	44,5	27,5	411	1	1	2	2
57,1 gr.	203,2 gr.	66,8 gr.	1591 kcal.	1798 kcal.	2011 kcal.	2552 kcal.	3000 kcal.

MEAL PLAN	TUESDAY	
BREAKFAST	*GARDEN GREEN SMOOTHIE*	1/2 Serving
A.M. SNACK	*MINI HAZELNUT DOUGHNUTS*	2 Servings
LUNCH	*QUICK QUINOA CASSEROLE*	2 Servings
P.M. SNACK	*PINEAPPLE SUNRISE SMOOTHIE*	1 Serving
DINNER	*CRUNCHY SESAME TOFU*	1 Serving
TOTAL		

FAT	CARBS	PROTEIN	CALORIES	SERVINGS	SERVINGS	SERVINGS	SERVINGS
12	25,2	14	264	1	1	1	1
19,6	5,6	9,6	237	2	2	2	2
22	49,8	18,4	470	2	2	3	3
2,3	60	2,9	272	1/2	1/2	1	1
20,9	17,7	16,9	326	1	1, 1/2	1, 1/2	3
76,8 gr.	158,3 gr.	61,8 gr.	1569 kcal.	1837 kcal.	1996 kcal.	2503 kcal.	2992 kcal.

MEAL PLAN	WEDNESDAY	
BREAKFAST	*EARLY MORNING OAT BUN*	1 Serving
A.M. SNACK	*TRAIL MIX ENERGY BAR*	1 Serving
LUNCH	*VEGGIEFUL' CHILI*	2 Servings
P.M. SNACK	*RASPBERRY CHEESECAKE*	1 Serving
DINNER	*MEXICAN CASSEROLE*	1/2 Serving
TOTAL		

FAT	CARBS	PROTEIN	CALORIES	SERVINGS	SERVINGS	SERVINGS	SERVINGS
12,7	30	9,4	271	1	1	2	2
10,4	44,9	7,2	302	1	1	1	1
9	87,2	26	512	2	2	2	3
23	8,2	5,6	262	1	2	2	2
5,5	27,9	10,1	221	1	1	1, 1/2	2
60,6 gr.	198,2 gr.	58,3 gr.	1568 kcal.	1789 kcal.	2051kcal.	2543kcal.	3020kcal.

MEAL PLAN	THURSDAY	
BREAKFAST	*BANANA-OAT CUPS*	1 Serving
A.M. SNACK	*NO-BAKE NUTELLA BARS*	1 Serving
LUNCH	*CREAMY CASHEW SPAGHETTI WITH ASPARAGUS*	1 Serving
P.M. SNACK	*MINI HAZELNUT DOUGHNUTS*	1 Serving
DINNER	*VEGAN FALAFEL BALLS*	6 Servings
TOTAL		

FAT	CARBS	PROTEIN	CALORIES	SERVINGS	SERVINGS	SERVINGS	SERVINGS
18	45	10,6	389	1	1	1	2
14,6	12,7	6,9	209	2	2	2	2
23,6	53,7	17	495	1	1	2	2
9,8	2,8	4,8	118	1	3	3	4
16,2	42	17,4	384	6	6	6	6
82,2 gr.	156,2 gr.	56,7 gr.	1595 kcal.	1804 kcal.	2040 kcal.	2535 kcal.	3042 kcal.

MEAL PLAN	FRIDAY	
BREAKFAST	*GARDEN GREEN SMOOTHIE*	1/2 Serving
A.M. SNACK	*BANANA BLUEBERRY MUFFINS*	1 Serving
LUNCH	*BLACK BEAN AND QUINOA BURRITO*	1 Serving
P.M. SNACK	*MEXIKALE CRIPS*	2 Servings
DINNER	*BAKED RED BELL PEPPERS*	2 Servings
TOTAL		

FAT	CARBS	PROTEIN	CALORIES	SERVINGS	SERVINGS	SERVINGS	SERVINGS
12	25,3	14	264	1	1	1	1
16,3	17,8	4,6	236	1	1	1	2
8,8	84	16,5	493	1	1	2	2
14,6	33,4	12	313	2	2	2	4
8	40	9	270	2	3	3	3
59,7 gr.	200,5 gr.	56,1 gr.	1577 kcal.	1842 kcal.	1977 kcal.	2470 kcal.	3019 kcal.

Week 3: Meal Plan

MEAL PLAN	MONDAY	
BREAKFAST	*BANANA OAT CUPS*	1 Serving
A.M. SNACK	*RASPBERRY LEMON ICE CREAM*	1 Serving
LUNCH	*BLACK BEAN SOUP*	2 Servings
P.M. SNACK	*ALMOND COOKIES*	3 Servings
DINNER	*CRUNCHY SESAME TOFU*	1 Serving
TOTAL		

FAT	CARBS	PROTEIN	CALORIES	SERVINGS	SERVINGS	SERVINGS	SERVINGS
18	45	10,6	389	1	1	1	1
17,5	8,3	1,8	198	2	2	2	3
17,8	58	19,4	470	2	2	4	4
18,6	5,1	3,9	231	3	6	6	6
20,9	17,7	17	327	1	1	1	2
92,8 gr.	134,1 gr.	52,7 gr.	1615 kcal.	1813 kcal.	2044 kcal.	2514 kcal.	3039 kcal.

MEAL PLAN	TUESDAY	
BREAKFAST	EARLY MORNING OAT BUN	1 Serving
A.M. SNACK	FLAXSEED YOGURT	1 Serving
LUNCH	COCONUT CURRY LENTIL SOUP	1/2 Serving
P.M. SNACK	NO-BAKE NUTELLA BARS	1 Serving
DINNER	BEAN BURRITOS	1 Serving
TOTAL		

FAT	CARBS	PROTEIN	CALORIES	SERVINGS	SERVINGS	SERVINGS	SERVINGS
12,7	30	9,4	271	2	2	2	3
16,9	9,2	10	220	1	1	1	1
25,5	45,3	14,5	467	1/2	1/2	1	1
14,6	12,7	6,9	209	1	1	1	1
11,4	76,2	14,5	408	1	1/2	1/2	2
81,1 gr.	173,4 gr.	55,3 gr.	1575 kcal.	1846 kcal.	2050 kcal.	2517 kcal.	2992 kcal.

MEAL PLAN	WEDNESDAY	
BREAKFAST	BERRY-BANA SMOOTHIE	1/2 Serving
A.M. SNACK	FLAXSEED YOGURT	1 Serving
LUNCH	SPICY BLACK BEAN SOUP WITH TORTILLA CHIPS	1/2 Serving
P.M. SNACK	PUMPKIN OAT MUFFINS	1 Serving
DINNER	TEMPEH CURRY	1 Serving
TOTAL		

FAT	CARBS	PROTEIN	CALORIES	SERVINGS	SERVINGS	SERVINGS	SERVINGS
5	83	3,5	391	1/2	1/2	1/2	1/2
16,9	9,2	10	220	2	3	3	3
17	55	10,4	414	1/2	1/2	1	1
2,8	22,8	3,6	130	1	1	2	2
13,7	44,5	27,5	411	1	1	1	2
55,4 gr.	214,5 gr.	55 gr.	1566 kcal.	1786 kcal.	2006 kcal.	2550 kcal.	2961 kcal.

MEAL PLAN		THURSDAY	
BREAKFAST	GARDEN GREEN SMOOTHIE		1/2 Serving
A.M. SNACK	TROPICAL CHIPS		1/2 Serving
LUNCH	CHICKPEA COUSCOUS		1 Serving
P.M. SNACK	MEXIKALE CRIPS		2 Serving
DINNER	SPICY BEET BOWL		1 Serving
TOTAL			

FAT	CARBS	PROTEIN	CALORIES	SERVINGS	SERVINGS	SERVINGS	SERVINGS
24	25,2	14	265	1/2	1/2	1/2	1/2
2,5	68,2	2,5	305	1/2	1/2	1	1
6	44,2	10	270	1	1	1	2
14,6	33,4	12	313	2	2	3	3
20,5	48,7	16,4	445	1, 1/2	2	2	2
67,6 gr.	219,7 gr.	54,9 gr.	1598 kcal.	1820 kcal.	2043 kcal.	2503 kcal.	3038 kcal.

MEAL PLAN		FRIDAY	
BREAKFAST	MATCHA MORNING BOWL		1 Servings
A.M. SNACK	PEACH-CAKE CHEESEBALL		1 Serving
LUNCH	EASY BABA GANOUSH		1 Serving
P.M. SNACK	MINI CHOCO-COCO CUPS		2 Servings
DINNER	VEGGIE POKE BOWL		1 Serving
TOTAL			

FAT	CARBS	PROTEIN	CALORIES	SERVINGS	SERVINGS	SERVINGS	SERVINGS
28	67,1	10,7	562	1	1	1	2
10,8	8	13,1	182	1	2	2	2
15,4	21,5	5,3	246	2	2	2	2
7,4	15,8	11,6	176	2	2	3	3
18,6	45,4	13,1	401	1	1	2	2
80,2 gr.	157,8 gr.	53,8 gr.	1567 kcal	1813 kcal.	1995 kcal.	2484 kcal.	3046 kcal.

Week 4: Meal plan

MEAL PLAN	MONDAY	
BREAKFAST	*ENERGY SMOOTHIE BOWL*	1/2 Serving
A.M. SNACK	*TRAIL MIX ENERGY BARS*	1 Serving
LUNCH	*MUSHROOM RAGOUT*	3 Servings
P.M. SNACK	*PEANUT BUTTER BROWNIES*	2 Servings
DINNER	*SPICY MEDITERRANEAN HUMMUS*	3 Servings
TOTAL		

FAT	CARBS	PROTEIN	CALORIES	SERVINGS	SERVINGS	SERVINGS	SERVINGS
12,3	54	5,1	347	1/2	1/2	1	1
10,4	44,9	7,2	302	1	1	1	2
12,3	12,6	7,5	231	6	9	9	9
17,6	12	20,4	284	2	2	2	3
23,4	39	15	411	3	3	4	4
76 gr.	162,5 gr.	55,2 gr.	1575 kcal.	1806 kcal.	2037 kcal.	2521 kcal.	2965 kcal.

MEAL PLAN		TUESDAY	
BREAKFAST	*DETOX SMOOTHIE BOWL*		1/2 Serving
A.M. SNACK	*BLUEBERRY ALMOND BITES*		2 Servings
LUNCH	*MEXICAN CASSEROLE*		1 Serving
P.M. SNACK	*NO-BAKE NUTELLA BARS*		1 Serving
DINNER	*ROASTED BELL PEPPER HUMMUS*		2 Servings
TOTAL			

FAT	CARBS	PROTEIN	CALORIES	SERVINGS	SERVINGS	SERVINGS	SERVINGS
1,2	60,1	0,5	250	1	1	1	2
34,4	12,2	25	452	2	2	4	4
11,5	65,9	20,2	442	1	1	1	1
14,6	12,7	6,9	209	1	2	2	2
6	26	9,2	194	2	2	2	2
67,7 gr.	176,9 gr.	61,8 gr.	1547 kcal.	1797 kcal.	2006 kcal.	2458 kcal.	2958 kcal.

MEAL PLAN		WEDNESDAY	
BREAKFAST	*BREAKFAST OATS BOWL*		1/3 Serving
A.M. SNACK	*PROTEIN PANCAKES*		2 Servings
LUNCH	*PUMPKIN PILAF*		1 Serving
P.M. SNACK	*ALMOND COOKIES*		3 Servings
DINNER	*SWEET POTATO CHICKPEA MINGLE*		1 Serving
TOTAL			

FAT	CARBS	PROTEIN	CALORIES	SERVINGS	SERVINGS	SERVINGS	SERVINGS
9,8	25,4	4,5	209	2/3	2/3	1	1
15,2	10,6	15,6	226	2	2	4	4
16,8	90,1	11,5	557	1	1	1	2
18,6	5,1	3,9	231	3	6	6	6
20,2	33,4	16	379	1	1	1	1
80,6 gr.	164,6 gr.	51,5 gr.	1602 kcal.	1811 kcal.	2042 kcal.	2477 kcal.	3034 kcal.

MEAL PLAN	THURSDAY	
BREAKFAST	PINEAPPLE SUNRISE SMOOTHIE	1/2 Serving
A.M. SNACK	MINI CHOCO-COCO CUPS	3 Servings
LUNCH	SWEET POTATO CURRY SOUP	1 Serving
P.M. SNACK	ALMOND COOKIES	4 Servings
DINNER	TEMPEH CURRY	1 Serving
TOTAL		

FAT	CARBS	PROTEIN	CALORIES	SERVINGS	SERVINGS	SERVINGS	SERVINGS
2,2	60	2,9	271	1/2	1/2	1/2	1/2
11,1	24,7	17,4	264	5	6	7	8
29,2	56,5	5	376	1	1	1	2
24,8	6,8	5,2	308	4	5	5	6
13,7	44,5	27,5	411	1	1	2	2
81 gr.	192,5 gr.	58 gr.	1630 kcal.	1806 kcal.	1971 kcal.	2460 kcal.	3001 kcal.

MEAL PLAN	FRIDAY	
BREAKFAST	BERRY-BANA SMOOTHIE	1/2 Serving
A.M. SNACK	PROTEIN PANCAKES	2 Servings
LUNCH	BBQ BEAN BOWL	2 Servings
P.M. SNACK	BANANA BLUEBERRY MUFFINS	1 Serving
DINNER	VEGAN FALAFEL BALLS	5 Servings
TOTAL		

FAT	CARBS	PROTEIN	CALORIES	SERVINGS	SERVINGS	SERVINGS	SERVINGS
5	83	3,5	391	1/2	1/2	1/2	1
15,2	10,6	15,6	226	2	2	2	3
20	50	12	430	2	2	4	4
16,3	17,8	4,6	236	1	1	1	1
13,5	35	14,5	320	5	8	8	8
70 gr.	196,4 gr.	50,2 gr.	1603 kcal.	1839 kcal.	2031 kcal.	2471 kcal.	2975 kcal.

Week 5: Meal Plan

MEAL PLAN	MONDAY	
BREAKFAST	*PEACHY MANGO BOWL*	1/2 Serving
A.M. SNACK	*MINI HAZELNUT DOUGHNUTS*	2 Servings
LUNCH	*CHEESY QUINOA*	2 Servings
P.M. SNACK	*PEACH-CAKE CHEESBALLS*	1 Serving
DINNER	*VEGGIEFUL CHILI*	1 Serving
TOTAL		

FAT	CARBS	PROTEIN	CALORIES	SERVINGS	SERVINGS	SERVINGS	SERVINGS
24,7	49,5	7,7	451	1/2	1/2	1	1
19,6	5,6	9,6	232	2	2	2	2
22,8	61,6	17,2	518	2	2	2	3
10,8	8	13,1	182	2	3	3	3
4,5	43,6	13	256	1	1	1	2
82,4 gr.	168,3 gr.	60,6 gr.	1639 kcal.	1821 kcal.	2003 kcal.	2454 kcal.	2969 kcal.

MEAL PLAN	TUESDAY	
BREAKFAST	*EARLY MORNING OAT BUN*	1 Serving
A.M. SNACK	*MAPLE SPELT COOKIES*	1 Serving
LUNCH	*WATERMELON SOY BOWL*	1 Serving
P.M. SNACK	*MINI CHOCO-COCO CUPS*	2 Servings
DINNER	*CHICKPEA COUSCOUS*	1 Serving
TOTAL		

FAT	CARBS	PROTEIN	CALORIES	SERVINGS	SERVINGS	SERVINGS	SERVINGS
12,7	30	9,4	271	1	1	1	2
15,2	42,4	8	338	1	1	2	2
27	58,5	12	525	1	1	1	1
7,4	15,8	11,6	176	2	4	6	8
6	44,2	10	270	2	2	2	2
68,3 gr.	190,9 gr.	51 gr.	1580 kcal.	1850 kcal.	2027 kcal.	2541 kcal.	2988 kcal.

MEAL PLAN	WEDNESDAY	
BREAKFAST	*GARDEN GREEN SMOOTHIE*	1/2 Serving
A.M. SNACK	*CHAI LATTE*	1 Serving
LUNCH	*BLACK BEAN AND QUINOA BURRITO*	1 Serving
P.M. SNACK	*PEANUT BUTTER BROWNIES*	1 Serving
DINNER	*SWEET POTATO CHICKPEA MINGLE*	1 Serving
TOTAL		

FAT	CARBS	PROTEIN	CALORIES	SERVINGS	SERVINGS	SERVINGS	SERVINGS
12	25,2	14	265	1/2	1	1	1
33,4	7,3	2,4	339	1	1	1	1
8,8	84	16,5	493	1	1	2	2
8,8	6	10,2	142	2	2	2	3
20,2	33,4	16	379	1	1	1	2
83,2 gr.	155,9 gr.	59,1 gr.	1618 kcal.	1760 kcal.	2025 kcal.	2518 kcal.	3039 kcal.

MEAL PLAN	THURSDAY	
BREAKFAST	*BANANA-OAT CUPS*	1 Serving
A.M. SNACK	*BLUEBERRY ALMOND BITES*	1 Serving
LUNCH	*ROASTED BEANS AND BASIL*	1 Serving
P.M. SNACK	*RASPBERRY CHEESCAKE*	1 Serving
DINNER	*BLACK BEAN BURGERS*	2 Serving
TOTAL		

FAT	CARBS	PROTEIN	CALORIES	SERVINGS	SERVINGS	SERVINGS	SERVINGS
18	45	10,6	389	1	1	1	2
17,2	6,1	12,5	226	1	1	1	1
32,4	11,9	4,9	338	1	1, 1/2	1, 1/2	2
23	8,2	5,6	262	1	1	2	2
6,4	72,4	19,8	414	3	3	4	4
97 gr.	143,6 gr.	53,4 gr.	1629 kcal.	1841 kcal.	2010 kcal.	2484 kcal.	3042 kcal.

MEAL PLAN	FRIDAY	
BREAKFAST	*MATCHA MORNING BOWL*	1/2 Serving
A.M. SNACK	*NO-BAKE NUTELLA BARS*	1 Serving
LUNCH	*VEGAN GOULASH*	1 Serving
P.M. SNACK	*PROTEIN PANCAKES*	2 Servings
DINNER	*RED CURRY LENTILS*	2 Serving
TOTAL		

FAT	CARBS	PROTEIN	CALORIES	SERVINGS	SERVINGS	SERVINGS	SERVINGS
14	33,5	5,3	281	1	1	2	3
14,6	12,7	6,9	209	2	2	3	3
18,7	83,8	16,5	591	1	1	1	1
15,2	10,6	15,6	226	2	2	2	4
13,6	38,6	12	324	2	3	3	3
76,1 gr.	179,2 gr.	56,3 gr.	1631 kcal.	1840 kcal.	2002 kcal.	2492 kcal.	2999 kcal.

Week 6: Meal Plan

MEAL PLAN	MONDAY	
BREAKFAST	*BREAKFAST PROTEIN BARS*	3 Servings
A.M. SNACK	*ENERGY SMOOTHIE BOWL*	1/2 Serving
LUNCH	*QUICK QUINOA CASSEROLE*	2 Serving
P.M. SNACK	*MEXIKALE CRIPS*	2 Servings
DINNER	*BLACK BEAN VEGGIE BURRITOS*	1 Serving
TOTAL		

FAT	CARBS	PROTEIN	CALORIES	SERVINGS	SERVINGS	SERVINGS	SERVINGS
12,9	7,8	11,4	183	6	6	6	6
12,3	54,1	5,1	347	1/2	1/2	1	1
22	29,8	18,4	472	2	3	3	5
14,6	33,4	12	313	2	2	3	3
9,8	40,9	8,6	285	1	1	1	1
71,6 gr.	166 gr.	55,5 gr.	1600 kcal.	1783 kcal.	2019 kcal.	2523 kcal.	2995 kcal.

MEAL PLAN	TUESDAY	
BREAKFAST	*MANGO BLASTER SMOOTHIE*	1/2 Serving
A.M. SNACK	*PEACH-CAKE CHEESEBALLS*	2 Servings
LUNCH	*QUINOA GREENS CASSEROLE*	2 Servings
P.M. SNACK	*MINI HAZELNUT DOUGHNUTS*	1 Serving
DINNER	*BAKED RED BELL PEPPERS*	2 Servings
TOTAL		

FAT	CARBS	PROTEIN	CALORIES	SERVINGS	SERVINGS	SERVINGS	SERVINGS
8,2	61	3,4	331	1/2	1/2	1	1, 1/2
21,6	16	26,2	364	3	3	3	4
29,2	54	17,8	550	2	2	2	2
9,8	2,8	4,8	116	1	3	3	3
8	40	9	270	2	2	3	3
76,8 gr.	173,8 gr.	61,2 gr.	1631 kcal.	1813 kcal.	2045 kcal.	2511 kcal.	3024 kcal.

MEAL PLAN	WEDNESDAY	
BREAKFAST	*BREAKFAST OATS BOWL*	1/3 Serving
A.M. SNACK	*PEACH CAKE CHEESEBALLS*	2 Servings
LUNCH	*CREAMY CASHEW SPHAGETTI WITH ASPARAGUS*	1 Serving
P.M. SNACK	*MAPLE SPELT COOKIES*	1 Serving
DINNER	*QUICK QUINOA CASSEROLE*	1 Serving
TOTAL		

FAT	CARBS	PROTEIN	CALORIES	SERVINGS	SERVINGS	SERVINGS	SERVINGS
9,8	25,4	4,5	209	1/3	2/3	2/3	1
21,6	16	26,2	364	3	3	3	3
23,6	53,7	17	495	1	1	2	2
15,2	42,4	8	338	1	1	1	1
11	24,9	9,2	236	1	1	1	2
81,2 gr.	162,4 gr.	64,9 gr.	1642 kcal.	1824 kcal.	2033 kcal.	2528 kcal.	2973 kcal.

MEAL PLAN	THURSDAY	
BREAKFAST	MANGO BLASTER SMOOTHIE	1/2 Serving
A.M. SNACK	BANANA BLUEBERRY MUFFINS	1 Serving
LUNCH	MEXICAN CASSEROLE	1 Serving
P.M. SNACK	PEANUT BUTTER BROWNIES	2 Servings
DINNER	TRIPLE BEAN CHILI	2 Servings
TOTAL		

FAT	CARBS	PROTEIN	CALORIES	SERVINGS	SERVINGS	SERVINGS	SERVINGS
8,2	61	3,4	331	1/2	1/2	1/2	1
16,3	17,8	4,6	236	2	2	2	2
11,5	65,9	20,2	442	1	1	2	2
17,6	12	20,4	284	2	2	3	3
7	46	11,8	286	2	3	3	4
60,6 gr.	202,7 gr.	60,4 gr.	1579 kcal.	1815 kcal.	1958 kcal.	2541 kcal.	3015 kcal.

MEAL PLAN	FRIDAY	
BREAKFAST	BERRY-BANA SMOOTHIE	1/2 Serving
A.M. SNACK	NO-BAKE NUTELLA BARS	1 Serving
LUNCH	QUINOA AND BROCCOLI STEW	1 Serving
P.M. SNACK	BLUEBERRY ALMOND BITES	1 Serving
DINNER	SPICY BEET BOWL	1 Serving
TOTAL		

FAT	CARBS	PROTEIN	CALORIES	SERVINGS	SERVINGS	SERVINGS	SERVINGS
5	83	3,5	391	1/2	1/2	1/2	1/2
14,6	12,7	6,9	209	2	2	2	3
10	47	12	326	1	1	1	2
17,2	6,1	12,5	226	1	2	2	2
20,5	48,7	16,4	445	1	1	2	2
67,3 gr.	197,5 gr.	51,3 gr.	1597 kcal.	1806 kcal.	2032 kcal.	2477 kcal.	3012 kcal.

SPICE RECIPES

Spice Ingredients

When it comes to making your food taste better, spices are an absolute must. They can drastically change and improve the overall taste of your meals and even contribute to a totally different flavor profile.

Spices can be changed according to personal taste and preference. If your shelf is abundant of spices, you will have the opportunity to get creative in the kitchen. By incorporating different spices, you can create a diversity of original tastes with the same recipes. It is good to know that there are both amazing and bad-tasting spice combinations. Choose a style of cooking and spicing up meals and products in order to create a matching flavor profile.

Knowing and learning spices will greatly improve your skills in the kitchen. Using and incorporating different seasoning combinations will guarantee unique twists to meals. This does not only go for complete meals but also to certain foods such as Hummus, nut-based milk products, plant-based cheeses, chickpea poppers and many other savory snacks

The spice recipes include the following ingredients:

- Nutritional yeast
- Ground turmeric
- Ground cumin
- Ground coriander
- Curry powder
- Chili powder

- Mustard powder
- Cardamom powder
- Garam masala
- Vanilla extract
- Black pepper
- Cayenne pepper

- Paprika
- Ground cinnamon
- Ground cloves
- Nutmeg
- Ground ginger

Recipes

BERBERE

This is an African spice made from:

- ½ cup chili powder or cayenne pepper
- ¼ cup sweet paprika
- 1 tbsp. salt
- ½ tsp. ground coriander
- 1 tsp. ground ginger
- ½ tsp. ground cardamom
- ½ tsp. ground fenugreek
- ¼ tsp. ground nutmeg
- 1/8 tsp. ground allspice
- 1/8 tsp. ground cloves.

DUKKAH

An Egyptian spice made from a mix of:

- 1 cup toasted nuts
- 1/3 cup sesame seeds
- 2/3 cup hazelnuts
- 3 tbsp. coriander
- 3 tbsp. cumin
- 1 tsp. ground pepper

HARISSA

A mixture of:

- 1 smoked red pepper
- ½ tsp. cumin
- ½ tsp. coriander
- ½ tsp. paprika
- 3 cloves garlic
- ½ tsp. sea salt
- ½ tsp. caraway
- 1 red onion

RAS EL HANOUT

A blend of:

- ¾ tsp. cumin
- ½ tsp. ginger
- ½ tsp. sea salt
- ½ tsp. black pepper
- 1¼ tsp. cinnamon
- ½ tsp. coriander
- ½ tsp. cayenne
- ¾ tsp. allspice

CHINESE FIVE SPICE

A mix of:

- 1 tsp. ground cinnamon
- 1 tsp. ground cloves
- ¼ tsp. fennel seed
- 1 tsp. star anise
- ¼ tsp. Szechuan peppercorns.

GOMASIO

A Japanese condiment that is a mix of:

- 2 cups toasted sesame seeds
- 1 tbsp. coarse salt

TOGARASHI

A mix of:

- 3 tbsp. chili pepper
- 3 tbsp. citrus peel
- 2 tbsp. sesame seeds
- 3 tbsp. Seaweed

FINES HERBES

A blend of fresh or dry herbs:

- 2 tbsp. chervil
- 2 tbsp. chives
- 4 tsps. tarragon
- 2 tbsp. parsley
- ½ tbsp. thyme
- 2 tbsp. chervil

KHMELI SUNELI

A Georgian mix of:

- 2 tsps. fenugreek
- 1 tbsp. coriander
- 1 tbsp. savory
- ½ tsp. black peppercorns.

QUATRE EPICES (FOUR SPICES)

A mix of:

- 2 tbsp. ground black and/or white pepper
- 1 tbsp. cloves
- 1 tbsp. nutmeg
- 1 tbsp. ginger.

CURRY POWDER

A mix of:

- ¼ cup turmeric
- 2 tbsp. coriander
- 2 tbsp. cumin
- 2 tbsp. fenugreek
- ½ tsp. red pepper.

PANCH PHORON

A mix of:

- 1 tbsp. fenugreek
- 1 tbsp. nigella
- 1 tbsp. cumin
- 1 tbsp. black mustard
- 1 tbsp. fennel seeds.

ADOBO

An all-purpose seasoning composed of:

- 1 tbsp. garlic
- 2 tbsp. oregano
- 3 tbsp. black pepper
- ¼ cup paprika
- 1 tbsp. garlic
- 2 tbsp. cumin

CHILI POWDER

A blend of:

- 1 tsp. ancho chili
- 2 tbsp. paprika
- 1¼ tsps. cumin
- 2 tsps. Mexican oregano.
- ¾ tsp. onion

JERK SPICE:

A spicy Jamaican composed of:

- 1 tsp. red and black pepper
- 1 tsp. allspice
- ¼ tsp. cinnamon
- 2 tsps. thyme
- 2 tsps. salt

ADVIEH

A mix of:

- 1 tsp. dried rose petals
- 1 tsp. cinnamon
- 1 tsp. cardamom
- 1 tsp. cloves
- 1 tsp. nutmeg
- ½ tsp. cumin

BAHARAT

A mixture of:

- 1 tsp. black pepper
- 2 tbsp. cumin
- ½ tsp. cinnamon
- ¼ tsp. cloves.
- ¼ tsp. cardamom
- 1 tsp. coriander

ZA'ATAR

A mix of:

- 2 tbsp. thyme
- 1 tbsp. sesame seeds
- ¼ cup sumac
- 2 tbsp. oregano
- 2 tbsp. marjoram

PICKLING SPICE

A blend of:

- 2 tbsp. bay leaves
- 2 tbsp. mustard seeds
- 1 tsp. peppercorns
- 2 tsps. coriander
- 1 tbsp. allspice

GARAM MASALA

A mix of:

- 2 tbsp. cinnamon
- 2 tbsp. cardamom
- 1 tbsp. cumin
- 2 tbsp. turmeric
- 1 tsp. mustard
- 1 tsp. fennel seed
- 2 red chilis

PUMPKIN PIE SPICE

A mix of:

- 4 tbsp. cinnamon
- ½ tsp. nutmeg
- 2 tbsp. ginger
- 1 tsp. cloves

MEXICAN SPICE

A blend of:

- 1 tablespoon cumin
- 1 tablespoon coriander
- 1 tablespoon paprika
- 1 teaspoon oregano
- 1/2 teaspoon chili
- 1/2 teaspoon garlic

CAJUN SPICE

A mixture of:

- 2 teaspoons salt
- 2 teaspoons garlic powder
- 2½ teaspoons paprika
- 1 teaspoon ground black pepper
- 1 teaspoon onion powder
- 1 teaspoon cayenne pepper
- 1¼ teaspoons dried oregano
- 1¼ teaspoons dried thyme
- ½ teaspoon red pepper flakes (optional)

Bonus

Welcome to the reader's circle of happyhealthygreen.life. You can subscribe to our newsletter using this link:

http://happyhealthygreen.life/vegan-newsletter

By subscribing to our newsletter, you will receive the latest vegan recipes, tips about health & nutrition and plant-based cooking articles that make your mouth water, right in your inbox. We also offer you a unique opportunity to read future vegan cookbooks for absolutely free...

Get your hands on free vegan recipes and instant access to 'The Vegan Cookbook'. Subscribe to the vegan newsletter and grab your free copy here at:

http://happyhealthygreen.life/vegan-newsletter

Enter your email address to get instant access. Support veganism and say NO to animal cruelty!

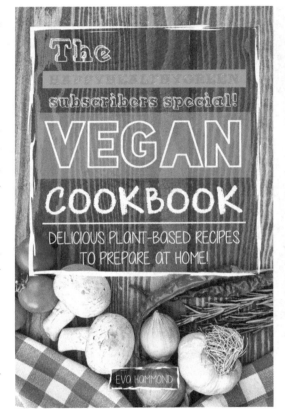

We don't like spam and understand you don't like spam either. We'll email you no more than 2 times per week.

Conclusion

Now that you have the necessary information and techniques to get started with meal prep, why not give it a try? There's nothing to lose – except excess weight – and if your goal is to live a healthier lifestyle, this practice will be of great benefit to you.

Meal prep enables you to have more control over the quantity and quality of the food you eat. All it takes is some planning and proper execution. You'll also save a lot of time in the kitchen, which is great -- especially if you don't like to cook.

We hope that this book has helped you on your way towards a healthier diet. Apply these concepts to get delicious and healthy prepared meals. Better yet, share what you have learned with others. This is an activity that can benefit you and your whole family.

Get started on meal prepping today. Take the knowledge in this book and make sure to shop for all the vegan ingredients you need. You will discover how food prep can change your life and your eating experience forever!

Thank you

Finally, if you enjoyed this book, then we would like to ask you for a small favor. Would you be kind enough to leave an honest review for this book? It'd be greatly appreciated by both the future reader and me!

You can send us your feedback here:

http://happyhealthygreen.life/about-us/jules-neumann/vegan-meal-prep1

Did you discover any grammar mistakes, confusing explanations or wrongful information? Don't hesitate to send us an email! You can reach us at **info@happyhealthygreen.life**

We promise to get back at you as soon as time allows us. If this book requires a revision, we'll send you the updated eBook for free after the revised book is available.

CPSIA information can be obtained
at www.ICGtesting.com
Printed in the USA
BVHW011230190819
556218BV00004B/28/P